WOMEN'S WORK,
WOMEN'S HEALTH

ALSO BY JEANNE MAGER STELLMAN

WORK IS DANGEROUS TO YOUR HEALTH
(with Susan M. Daum, M.D.)

WOMEN'S WORK, WOMEN'S HEALTH

Myths and Realities

BY
JEANNE MAGER STELLMAN

With illustrations by Lyda Pola

PANTHEON BOOKS, NEW YORK

All rights reserved under International and Pan-American
Copyright Conventions. Published in the United States by
Pantheon Books, a division of Random House, Inc., New York,
and simultaneously in Canada by Random House of Canada
Limited, Toronto.

Library of Congress Cataloging in Publication Data

Stellman, Jeanne M., 1947–
Women's Work, Women's Health.

Bibliography: p. 245
Includes index.
1. Industrial hygiene—United States.   2. Women—
Health and hygiene—United States.   3. Women—Employment
—United States.   4. Occupational diseases.   5. Women—
Diseases. I. Title. [DNLM: 1. Women. 2. Employment.
3. Health.   WA491 S824w]
RC963.7.U6S73   613.6'2   77-5200
ISBN 0-394-73452-1 pbk.
ISBN 0-394-41038-6

Grateful acknowledgment is made to the following for permission to reprint from previously published material:

The New York Times: Brief quotation of Flossie Strickland from
an article in the May 15, 1977, issue of *The New York Times* by
B. Drummond Ayres, Jr. Copyright © 1977 by the New York
Times Company. Reprinted by permission.

Wall Street Journal: Excerpts from an article in the February 5,
1976, issue of the *Wall Street Journal* by John O'Riley. Copyright © 1977 by Dow Jones & Company, Inc.

Manufactured in the United States of America

FIRST EDITION

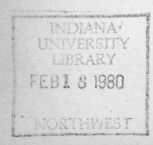

To Sam and Mandy Stellman
for the way they taught their son.

Contents

List of Illustrations

ILLUSTRATIONS

List of Tables

Acknowledgments

IT IS DIFFICULT to acknowledge the people and events that helped formulate this book. It has been only five or six years since a number of us, socially conscious science and health professionals, formed the Scientists' Committee for Occupational Health and taught a course for workers on health and safety at the Rutgers Labor Education Center. Out of that experience came the book *Work Is Dangerous to Your Health* and the re-orientation of several careers from pure science to occupational health. For this change I must acknowledge and thank Tony Mazzocchi. The Oil, Chemical and Atomic Workers International Union provided the training ground for me, and I especially want to thank Al Grospiron, president, and Tony Sabatine, secretary-treasurer, for their faith that a young female scientist could do the job.

Without Sylvia Krekel our work at the Union would have been stymied. She is also a good friend. Finally the rank-and-file, their lives, perceptions, and problems were an important formative part of the experiences that went into making up this book.

The gap between general occupational health and women's occupational health was in part bridged by the rather prejudiced assumption made by so many people that as a woman I would automatically understand "women's problems." So I must acknowledge that erroneous assumption, which forced me to learn and research the area in order to prepare the speeches and lectures I was asked to give.

In a more positive vein there are a few women whom I wish particularly to acknowledge: Vilma Hunt, for her help, her enthusiasm, her talent, her work (and her example of coping with the dual role of homemaker and worker); Kathleen O'Leary, for her knowledge and interest; Andrea Hricko, for helping to create a movement; Odessa Komer, for her steadfastness and support; Clara Schiffer, for her eternal optimism and effort.

Barbara Wertheimer and Anne Nelson, of the Women's Trade Union Program at Cornell in New York City, allowed me the opportunity to develop and teach some of my thoughts to their wonderful worker-students. Working with the Coalition of Labor Union Women's Occupational Safety and Health Task Force on their testimony before OSHA on the proposed lead-exposure standard gave me the opportunity to learn how important it is for the women's movement to be vigilant and united. Anne Trebilcock, Geri Palast, Ellen Hall, Pam Schnierle, Gloria Gordon, and Joan Graff deserve special thanks. I wish to thank Sid Stone for the *Harper's Weekly* illustration.

Perhaps the most important force in this book has been my editor, Susan Gyarmati. She tolerated handwritten outlines and barely legible copy, helped me nurture the ideas, patiently (at times) criticized, and read and re-read the pages. Her perceptions, enthusiasm, and encouragement were absolutely essential and are deeply appreciated. Donna Grusky Bass has also played an essential role, and I thank her for it and for her almost superhuman concentration. Carol Lazare has been, as always, tremendously helpful.

I must also acknowledge my husband, who—although he did *not* do the typing—has of his own accord shared so many of the duties of home and family that it was possible for me to write this book. Martha Gary also must be thanked. Without her help at home, my options and opportunities would have been very limited. And finally, I wish to acknowledge the two severe cases of tonsillitis that our children, Andrew and Emma, developed just as all the deadlines approached. They made me realize once again just how tenuous is the ability of women to successfully combine employment, home, and family in our society today.

Foreword

SEVERAL YEARS AGO I was reading an article in the U. S. Department of Labor publication *Job Safety and Health*. In that article, which dealt with the occupational safety and health hazards faced by women workers, I read a quote by Jeanne Stellman, in which she predicted that the jobs of many women workers would be threatened and lost because of what industry feared were potential adverse effects of their working conditions on their ability to produce healthy children. In order to avoid any adverse effects from occurring, industry would simply eliminate women from "hazardous" jobs, Stellman said. Well, at that time I thought to myself that this woman was an alarmist, another doomsayer and pessimist. After all, with Title VII opening up all sorts of new opportunities for women and offering protections against discrimination in the workplace, what could this new form of discrimination really amount to?

Then in December 1975, General Motors Corporation of Canada eliminated women of childbearing age from employment in the storage-battery operation in the shop where there was exposure to lead. The women were moved right out unless they could prove to the satisfaction of the company that they could not have children. And so I found out that the predictions made by Jeanne Stellman were not alarmist—they are coming true, and we in the trade-union movement and other movements are faced with some severe problems.

Over the last decade, women workers have seen a slow but steady improvement in the job opportunities available to them. Women have just begun to gain access, during a period of peacetime production, to exclusively male enclaves of work. With the suggestion of an exclusionary policy, we see a throwback to the definition of women as homemaker and secondary worker. But most women do not want to be restricted to these roles. Among other considerations, they do not pay well. Most women workers seek and hold jobs for the same reasons men do. About three-quarters of all working women either support themselves and/or their families alone, or work to bring their family income above $10,000 a year, an amount now inadequate to maintain even middle-class life. Forcing women out of their jobs will only bring economic hardship to more Americans.

Thus, women are faced with a number of contradictory situations. Every time I read the newspaper or listen to the news I hear of some new environmental disaster—which usually means that harm to the fetus is also predicted. But the headlines go beyond disaster situations to situations more commonly occurring. According to some experts, for example, caffeine may damage a fetus; noise may be injurious to a fetus; other chemicals, heat, and so on may all have adverse effects. If the pattern set by the lead industry were to be followed by other employers, virtually every woman's job would be in jeopardy, since so many women encounter some sort of potential hazard while they work.

On the other hand, if there are potential hazards which cannot be removed, it is also important to realize that simply excluding those persons perceived of as more vulnerable still allows others to remain exposed to toxic conditions. Thus, a policy of exclusion of fertile women from lead-exposure jobs will not help women, or men, or their unborn children. Only standards set at a level to protect all workers will truly serve the aims of our society as enunciated by the Occupational Safety and Health Act (OSHA). For the purpose of OSHA is clear: "to assure so far as possible *every* working man and woman in the nation safe and healthful working conditions and preserve our human resources."

Another contradiction arises, however, when we consider the alternatives available to a woman who works in an environment that may be unsafe and who wants to avoid any risks. Just recently automatic eligibility for temporary income-replacement plans for maternity-related disabilities was disallowed by the U. S. Supreme Court. Such a benefit was part of Title VII of the Civil Rights Act and provided the same disability pay for pregnant women that any other worker is entitled to when he or she is temporarily unable to work. If women cannot have economic backup when they do wish to work because they may be exposed to something injurious to their fetuses while they are pregnant, and also are not allowed the option to continue to work, what then are their real choices? Even people that become pregnant have to eat.

Recently the United Auto Workers and others have urged the United States Congress to extend the provisions of Title VII, which prohibits discrimination in the workplace, to explicitly disallow discrimination on the basis of pregnancy. This would insure that temporary work-disability benefit programs be applied to pregnancy-related work disability. The UAW has already negotiated such benefits for some of its female members in its contracts. We told the Congress that those companies that set up disability programs for pregnancy did not encounter the economic debacle that was widely predicted. Several companies—and not the very largest and richest—have found the maternity benefit actually to be an inconsequential cost of the total employee benefits package.

Part of the reason that the untrue predictions of huge costs ignore some of the realities about women is that they are based on false stereotypes. They ignore the fact that many women delay employment until after completing childbearing. They are based on the belief that women would abuse disability and would malinger, a charge that is without foundation and that is fundamentally insulting to women. Since the disability would have to be certified by a physician, with the provision that if the company physician disagreed, a third physician could be brought in, which effectively defeats that argument, the "malingering" charge boils down to a perpetuation of unjust stereotypes about women workers—one being that women take no fundamental interest in their jobs or careers and hence would always malinger if given the opportunity.

In this book, this and many of the other stereotypes about women, their work, and their health are discussed—and it always seems to come down to the same thing—the myths and the realities don't coincide. And too often, the myths about women end up forcing women to choose between their jobs and their health.

It is interesting that many of the same elements in our society that would seek to deny women Aid to Dependent Children or other public assistance when they and their children are in need are the same people who would deny a woman her job—or her right to return to one—because of the possibility of damage to her fetus, even if she doesn't plan to bear children. There has to be some middle road, some rationality. It is not difficult to find the path down that road. The accepted reality is that women—and men— need a workplace that is safe from recognized hazards. That is their right under the Occupational Safety and Health Act of 1970. They need the right to earn a living and still retain the capacity to bear healthy children. What they need is a job that is safe enough for a fetus—and safe enough for its parents.

If women are to gain their rights to working and maintaining their health and safety, they must understand the potential problems that they are facing. For too long we have lived with stereotypes like the assumption that just because a woman is capable of bearing children, she will. *Women's Work, Women's Health* helps us to unravel the truth, and helps us to separate the myths from the realities.

—Odessa Komer
Vice President, UAW

WOMEN'S WORK,
WOMEN'S HEALTH

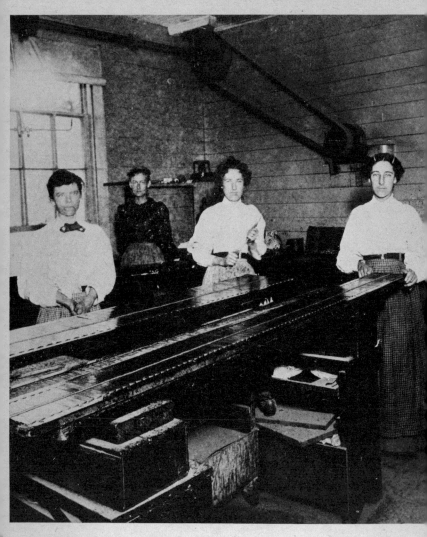

The four young women in this late-nineteenth-century shop were employed in the manufacture of metal objects like rules, planes, gauges, screws, and doorstops. They were exposed to the toxic, perhaps deadly, fumes of the molten metal as it was cast in dies. Their workplace was unventilated; their working hours, long.

CREDIT: The Connecticut Historical Society

CHAPTER ONE
BOUND BY CONCEPTION

If the income brought into family coffers by the womenfolk of the country were suddenly cut off, the nation's high flying "standard of living" would collapse overnight. . . . The close of 1975 saw more adult women at work than ever before. . . . The workingman breadwinner who doesn't have a wife on a payroll just may wind up not having enough bread.

—John O'Riley
The Wall Street Journal
February 5, 1976

IN 1976 IT WAS front-page news in the nation's leading business newspaper that women work. It was apparently even greater news that women workers make an essential contribution to the economy. A new image of an income-producing working wife is replacing the old image of a child-producing housewife. And faced with nearly a majority of the adult females already actively participating in the economy, those in the business of studying human behavior and trends are naturally trying to explain this "phenomenon"—they want to know why women are working.

The very need for an explanation arises from the implicit assumption that nature defines a woman as a wife, a childbearer, and a homemaker, and not as a contributor to economic life. If modern women do become economically active, this must be "explained." Explanations are sought that revolve around the biological role of childbearing and the physical role of homemaking, so as to be consistent with nature's supposed definition of woman. Thus, the theory for the current increase in the number of women in the workplace is based on the premises that because the modern small family makes child rearing easier, and because modern medicine makes life easier and longer, women are now free to go to work.

The pieces seem to fit together, and the theory represents the conventional wisdom on the subject of why women are working. It is aptly summarized in the following statement:

> A series of technological and business innovations early in the century provided less costly substitutes for the manual work performed by women in the home. Perhaps even more significant was the dramatic change in child-related aspects of a woman's life. For example, in 1910 married women in the age group of 45 to 59 years had borne an average of five children; by 1950 the number of children borne had declined to about half that figure. Notable among the factors contributing to this decrease in births was the decline in infant and child mortality, which meant fewer births were needed to achieve a given desired family size. The spread of birth control information also had an important impact. The span of years during which women could work continuously was lengthened by declines in their mortality combined with the completion of the childbearing period at an earlier age. Increases in their number of years of schooling and greater urbanization were other factors adding to the pull from the home to the marketplace.[1]

The theoretical structure is thus that fewer children and less housework have "pulled" women from the home. This structure seems sound—until its underpinnings are examined. A careful review of the statistics related to birth and death, and of the participation of women as workers in the twentieth century, just does not support these arguments. Birth-rate data show that from at least 1910–1960, the majority of women gave birth to no children or to only one or two live-born children during their lifetimes. This majority could easily have been employed outside the home if it were the burdens of childbearing that were the major constraint keeping them from work. In fact, however, since

1960 the growth in the numbers of women returning to economic activity has occurred at the same time that more women are raising families than at any other period during this century. As will be shown, the vast majority of women now are mothers of at least two children, and childlessness is rapidly disappearing.

Similarly, while there have been declines in the death rate throughout the twentieth century, and consequently a greater life expectancy, neither factor explains the increase in female work-force participation, since, as we will see, the life expectancy of the twentieth-century woman has been long enough to permit decades of productive economic life, even if she did opt to devote many years solely to bearing and raising a family.

Furthermore, contrary to popular belief, the span of years devoted to childbearing has essentially remained the same throughout this century, ending for most childbearing women by the age of 35—an age certainly young enough to allow for many years of work outside the home.

The arguments of easier homemaking can be refuted when we see that the home today, replete with mechanical gadgetry, demands as much time of women now as it did of their grandmothers two generations ago. Similarly, standards of mothering have changed. Women are bombarded with theories of child development that often cause them to question their own instincts and doubt their own abilities to raise their children. Women have become master chefs, sanitarians, and psychologists, so that if more and more women are returning to work, it is not because society has provided them with nothing else to fill their time.

When these arguments are combined with the fact that in the past ten years the largest percentage increase of women working has been among mothers of young children, who have the greatest home and child responsibilities, we see that differences in childbearing and child-rearing patterns, longevity, and homemaking cannot explain why women are going to work. The generalizations about woman's place and woman's biological functions are not true. They are based on misread statistics, inadequate data, and an adamant refusal to recognize the economic value of woman's work and even her very existence as a worker. It is the purpose of this book to examine the status of women as workers, and to present material on the relationships between women and their work and health.

The Case of Careful Concealment

Before the Industrial Revolution, women played a vital and acknowledged role in the mainstream of Western economic life, which was, of course, centered around the home and the land. In agrarian England, for example, male wage earners were usually paid only enough to support themselves, because it was assumed their wives would be supporting the rest of the family.[2] Or, another example, from 1743:

> Consider, my dear girl, that you have no portions, and endeavour to supply the deficiencies of fortune of mind. You cannot expect to marry in such a manner, as neither of you shall have occasion to work, and none but a fool will take a wife whose bread must be earned solely by his labour and who will contribute nothing towards it herself.[3]

The life and times were hard, but men and women openly shared the burden.

The changes wrought by industrialization slowly and continually squeezed women out of the economic mainstream. Urban living made farming impossible; and the domestic industries, largely textile, were destroyed by the competition of mass production. The eradication of home industries created a major problem for the large percentage of women who were unmarried. The figures in 1911, for example, indicated that 46 percent of the women of working age were unmarried, with another 9.2 percent widowed.

The great majority of these women were working to support themselves.

Before industrialization such women had generally earned their living by spinning, the origin of the term "spinster." Of the few industries in existence, like dairy and brewing, only some were also open to women. But the unmarried or widowed working-class woman during the early industrial era no longer had the option of home industry. She was forced to enter industry in one of the low-paid factory jobs, like textile or laundry work, or else she could become a servant. The literature of the period, such as Dickens's *Hard Times,* is replete with tales of horror about the conditions of women and children at work during those times. And the unmarried middle-class woman did not fare any better. When thrown on her own resources, although she was spared the factory, she was usually forced to become a governess, at even lower wages and subject to degrading working conditions well documented in the novels of Charlotte Brontë and others. Yet, despite the large number of women working, the role of the woman worker became less recognized as industry "progressed."

The powerful image of the woman as preserver of home and hearth that grew along with industrialization has managed to obscure the role of woman as wage earner. So deeply ingrained are the myths about women that it is startling to examine the statistics of the large number of women at work between 1870 and 1930, which are summarized in Table 1a.

Twenty percent of the female population was employed outside the home at the turn of the century. These figures are an underestimate because women who labored on farms are underrepresented. While the census data show almost half the male population engaged in agricultural work between 1870 and 1900, less than 4 percent of the women were recorded as so employed. This is because farmers' wives and older daughters who toiled on the family farm

TABLE 1a. WOMEN WORKERS IN THE TWENTIETH CENTURY

WOMEN WORKERS AND THEIR OCCUPATIONS, 1870–1930

Occupations	1930	1920	1910	1900	1890	1880	1870
Total number	10,752,116	8,636,512	7,444,787	5,319,397	4,005,532	2,647,157	1,917,446
Agriculture	909,939	1,170,147	1,175,639	1,008,365	795,979	625,849	454,944
Forestry and fishing	329	673	557	687	324	65	36
Extraction of minerals	759	2,864	1,094	1,269	545	132	56
Manufacturing and mechanical industries	1,886,307	1,930,352	1,820,847	1,380,469	1,047,968	657,762	364,097
Transportation and communication	281,204	224,270	115,347	42,181	17,605	3,676	1,050
Trade	962,680	671,983	472,703	297,966	141,593	57,032	18,735
Public service (not elsewhere classified)	17,583	10,586	4,836	3,198	1,643	672	145
Professional service	1,526,234	1,017,030	734,752	436,174	312,747	176,824	94,166
Domestic and personal service	3,180,251	2,186,682	2,530,403	1,962,035	1,610,068	1,118,105	982,307
Clerical occupations	1,986,830	1,421,925	588,609	187,053	77,060	7,040	1,910

PERCENT DISTRIBUTION

Occupations	1930	1920	1910	1900	1890	1880	1870
Agriculture	8.5	13.5	15.8	19.0	19.9	23.6	23.7
Forestry and fishing	—	—	—	—	—	—	—
Extraction of minerals	—	—	—	—	—	—	—
Manufacturing and mechanical industries	17.5	22.4	24.5	26.0	26.2	24.8	19.0
Transportation and communication	2.6	2.6	1.5	0.8	0.4	0.1	0.1
Trade	9.0	7.8	6.3	5.6	3.5	2.2	1.0
Public service (not elsewhere classified)	0.2	0.1	0.1	0.1	—	—	—
Professional service	14.2	11.8	9.9	8.2	7.8	6.7	4.9
Domestic and personal service	29.6	25.3	34.0	36.9	40.2	42.2	51.2
Clerical occupations	18.5	16.5	7.9	3.5	1.9	0.3	0.1

SOURCE: U. S. Bureau of the Census, *16th Census Comparative Statistics* (Washington, D.C., 1943).

1b) DISPARITY BETWEEN PERCENTAGES OF MALES AND FEMALES
RECORDED IN AGRICULTURAL PURSUITS

Adjusted percent of women employed, 1870–1930: An arbitrary addition of one half the difference between male and female workers in the agricultural work-force participation is added to the number and percent of females employed to derive the following figures, which may be a better reflection of, true female work-force participation.

	% Agricultural Workers		Corrected		% Total Females Employed
	Males	Females	%	#	
1930	21.6	1.9	21.6	5,286,720	36.1
1920	26.3	2.8	23.5	4,806,448	35.4
1910	30.3	3.3	27.0	4,908,897	37.5
1900	36.3	3.4	32.9	4,660,201	37.0
1890	41.6	3.2	38.4	4,255,310	38.2
1880	47.7	3.3	44.2	3,759,287	38.2
1870	50.4	3.3	47.1	3,101,752	30.1

were generally not considered gainfully employed in agriculture, while the owner of the farm—the husband and father—was. As agricultural employment declined for men and women, both sexes had to seek employment in industry.

Before the beginning of World War II, the figure for the female population employed outside the home had practically reached 30 percent. World War II, with its expanded opportunities and encouragement for female employment, brought the work-force level to 38 percent of all women. And despite the baby boom, which followed the war, and the pressures of women to leave the workplace to make room for the returning soldiers, the percent of employed women has not again dropped below the 30 percent level, as Figure 1 shows.

Nonetheless, the doors of industry have not swung open for women as they have for men. Women also have not entered diversified occupations the way that men have, as we will see in greater detail in the next chapter. The major expansion of women workers has been in the area of clerical work; but as Figure 10 in the next chapter shows,

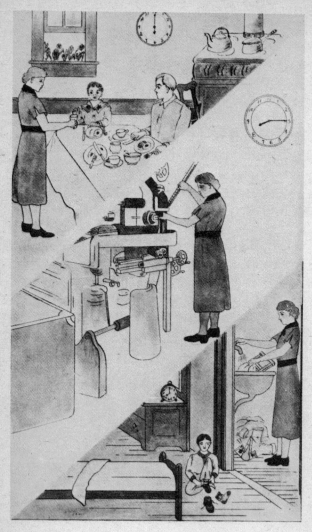

Illustration 1. THE DUAL ROLE OF WOMEN

The dual role of work at home and work on the job is not new.

SOURCE: U. S. Department of Labor Women's Bureau, *The Employed Woman Homemaker in the United States,* Women's Bureau Bulletin no. 148 (Washington, D. C., 1936).

the percentage of all jobs that clerical work represents has remained consistently low. For women workers, however, clerical work is now the major area of employment. The graphs in Figure 10 show this clearly. Less than one out of every six jobs is a clerical job, but it represents work for about one out of every three women. Thus, women have been joining the ranks of a huge clerical army that does not represent an expansion of economic growth but rather an expansion of paper overflow: three out of every four clerical workers is a woman.

The Leisured Woman

There were, of course, many women who did not contribute their labor to the economy. The Industrial Revolution created an entirely new class of people—the middle class. For the first time in history, substantial numbers of men could earn enough money to support a wife and family without the labor of the wife. The "leisured woman" became a symbol of the newly acquired affluence of the middle class. Her leisure was testimony to her husband's success. She represented the security of home and hearth, a retreat from the ugliness of business.

> The man . . . must encounter all peril and trial; to him, therefore, must be the failure, the offence, the inevitable error; often he must be wounded, or subdued; often misled, and *always* hardened. But he guards the woman from all this; within his house, as ruled by her, unless she herself has sought it, need enter no danger, no temptation, no cause of error or offence. This is the true nature of home— it is the place of Peace; the shelter, not only from all injury, but from all terror, doubt, and division.[4]

The leisured Victorian lady was forbidden to work, think, vote, sign contracts, or even automatically gain custody of her children if her husband died. The work of homemaking, as well as any other useful occupation, was denied her. Her home and children were given over to the multitudes of available servants, eager for work. However,

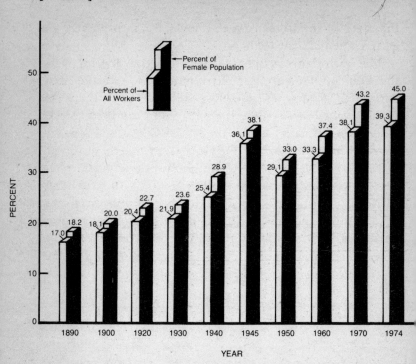

Figure 1. PERCENTAGE OF WOMEN IN THE LABOR FORCE, 1890–1974
The percentage of women employed is an underestimate, at least until 1930, because farm women were generally not counted as employed, while their husbands were (see Table 1).

SOURCE: U.S. Department of Labor Women's Bureau, *1975 Handbook on Women Workers* (Washington, D.C., 1975).

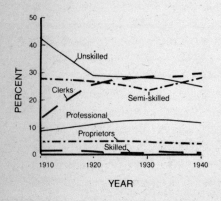

Figure 1b shows that the major expansion of jobs has been into clerical positions and not into skilled and professional areas.

SOURCE: U.S. Bureau of the Census, *16th Census: Population Comparative Statistics for the United States, 1870–1940* (Washington, D.C., 1943).

the myth of the woman on the pedestal was promptly forgotten when it came to the working woman.

The Victorian era thus created a new burden for working women. Not only were they forced to leave the home and enter low-paying, alienating jobs to make their economic contributions, but the very fact that they worked made them socially undesirable. The social (and legal, as we shall see) pressures on working women were enormous. As relative affluence spread to the working class, many heretofore working women began retreating from the workplace into the home, even if their budgets and their sense of self-fulfillment could have profited from continued participation in the labor force. For the woman who supported herself and possibly her family, the scorn and mistreatment of her was particularly difficult.

The Motherhood Myth

The leisured-women image of middle-class women created a major psychological obstacle to their economic participation. A second one was also created by the mythologizing of motherhood. It became the sacred duty of women to be perfect mothers, inspiring and guiding their offspring. "A woman when she becomes a mother should withdraw herself from the world, devote herself to her child."[5] But while the sanctity of motherhood was thus declared, the actual tasks of mothering were given over to nurses, governesses, and boarding schools. The middle-class woman indeed spent very little time with her children, often even hiring a wet nurse to feed her newly born infant. The accepted mark of affluence was a nursery maid for each child.

Despite the contradictions between the theory and the practice of Victorian motherhood, its mythology became so well rooted that dire spectres of neglected, delinquent children were consistently raised as arguments against the employment of women. So sacred had motherhood become that the large number of women who did not bear children were usually thought to be remiss in attending to those duties within the proper sphere of women. They were incomplete females.

A classic illustration of the twentieth-century "incomplete" working female is the career woman in the movies who is saved from her dire fate by wedding the male protagonist, just as Katharine Hepburn was duly rescued by Spencer Tracy in *Woman of the Year*. We may sit back and smile at that movie today, but we really have not escaped from the Tracy-Hepburn complex. Although many young women may expect to pursue careers or to combine work outside the home with raising families, most women still do not prepare themselves for lives as successful self-supporting wage earners or career women. Their education and training are almost universally self-limiting, restricting them to relatively low-paying "woman's work" with little chance for upward mobility or diversification. Further, whatever the *expectation*, marriage and family are the *actual* experience for the vast majority of women.

The psychological barriers to women working today are much more subtle than those that were prevalent during the Victorian era or the Tracy-Hepburn days. Although the choice for women is no longer between career and family, the current perceptions of women "making it" reflect neither the reality of the psychological and social burdens that women bear nor the barriers to combining work with raising a family. Whenever young mothers share their experiences, they find that guilt and concern over the welfare of their children and the effects of working on the child's development are major emotional burdens. This is particularly true when there are so many psychologists and other social scientists busy observing the young and "pinpointing" the most crucial periods of child development.

The accuracy with which some observers are apparently able to determine these most crucial moments in childhood development is almost awesome. We have progressed from the concepts of the critical first five years of life to the critical first three years to the critical first three months and now even to the critical first weeks of a child's life. As it is noted that small infants do indeed perceive their environments to a far greater extent than had been "officially" realized before, it is often solemnly declared that the environment during this time is crucial and may determine the future well-being of the child. These declarations are published in popular books and magazines, and are well circulated among women.

While it is undoubtedly true that very young children do perceive a great deal about their environment (which most observant mothers knew in the first place), there is no substantiation that the continual presence of a mother is necessary for a child's health. It most certainly cannot be necessary for a mother's health, since the unrelieved companionship of one's offspring can become unbearable. There has been no scientific confirmation that the children of working mothers suffer in any measurable emotional, social, or intellectual way. In fact, scientists have been unable to develop any positive or negative correlation between social and psychological parameters of children and the employment of their mothers.

We also know very little about the long-range effects of the absence of fathers and other close relatives on the child's development. Before the modern industrial era, many children, especially in rural settings, were raised in close contiguity to male parents and to the extended family. It might be worthwhile for social scientists to explore these questions of potential social deprivation so that the burdens of guilt can be shared more equitably.

Whatever the scientific reality, the sociological fact is that child raising is the female's responsibility in modern society. And while the Industrial Revolution has resulted in the urbanization of the population, the dissolution of the extended family, and the virtual removal of the father from the parenting role, it has not resulted in alternative social methods for aiding women in the role of parent. Child-care and work arrangements suitable to the demands of family, home, and work are virtually nonexistent.

The rapid reversal of norms that is occurring has shattered the image of the leisured woman, and the recognized sphere of women is quickly being moved from the home to the marketplace. Women are facing the expectation of working outside the home at the same time that their household work remains unrecognized and uncompensated. They are often expected to assume the dual obligations of home and job, and the economics of many modern families depend on two paychecks. As we will see, however, just as the social programs for helping women cope with two workplaces have not grown, neither have the opportunities in the marketplace for better and more satisfying jobs expanded.

One extreme response to the awesome burden of two full-time jobs is the popularized "total woman"—a new glorification of women in their home role which is a modern version of the Victorian leisured woman with the sex taboo removed. The total woman—sexually vibrant, always eager and enthusiastic about home, family, and husband—no more represents the real joys and dilemmas of modern women than the leisured woman represented the realities of the Victorian era.

The Dilemma of the Dual Role

While the rights of women to meaningful participation in the work force are clear and should not be discouraged, at the same time the difficulties of combining the work of the home and the work of outside employment should not be underestimated. When the home industries were taken from women, so too was their identity as workers in the home. The rapid, massive industrial production of goods and services led to a redefinition of work in terms of market value in trade rather than in terms of expended human labor or human social needs. Since the work performed by most women in the home was not bartered, bought, or sold, it bore no defined market value; hence, it soon ceased to be considered work. Women are still in the same position, which is further buttressed by the market value accorded to work performed by women hired for housework. Private household workers were, and continue to be, among the lowest paid of all workers, although some of their skills can be compared to higher-paid industrial workers.

A woman's household duties require long hours of labor each week and consist of many tasks that are disagreeable, monotonous, and unchallenging—all characteristics of stressful work. Further, sociologist Ann Oakley's studies of housework, as well as other related surveys, confirm the truth of the old saying that "woman's work is never done." Women today spend as much or more time engaged in housework as their grandmothers did. Housework is a job that covers a seven-day week, fifty-two weeks a year. Most of the women surveyed by Oakley spent at least seventy hours per week engaged in household chores. This represents an increase of about six hours of work per week over the time spent by rural housewives two decades earlier.[6]

Part of the increase in housework time results from changes in the levels of expectation. People own more clothes, which are kept cleaner because of washing machines, which in turn have created more laundry and higher standards of "cleanliness." Larger houses, more possessions, more household gadgets to use, as well as the availability of fresh food year round, have increased the work load for women and have raised the standards for being a "good housewife." The pressures of advertisement and the conceptions of ideal family life as portrayed on television present strong social pressures on women to conform to these arbitrary standards. The cleanliness of the toilet bowl, the shine on the floor, and the pinkness of baby's bottom are all criteria that have been set by advertising slogans and the inventiveness of consumer marketing, and that add to the house worker's burden. Some of the data on housework obligations and practices are summarized in Table 2.

Betty Friedan has aptly noted that housework expands to fill the time allotted to it,[7] and we have just seen that indeed there are excesses to current conceptions of "good housekeeping"; but one should not overlook the fact that housework *is* work. Even if a woman is not a gourmet cook, superb housekeeper, or extravagant decorator, she is still obligated to spend hours shopping and running household errands, doing laundry and cooking and cleaning, even for just minimal household management.

It is interesting to note that many of the shopping tasks that women face today are a direct result of the mechanization of industry, which made the production of goods and services in the home, particularly textiles, less economic than the purchasing of ready-made items. Also, the urbanization of the population made the raising, canning, and preserving of family foods impossible, so that this avenue

TABLE 2. A COMPARISON OF DATA ON HOUSEWORK HOURS

STUDY	DATE	AVERAGE WEEKLY HOURS OF HOUSEWORK
Rural Studies		
United States	1929	63
United States	1956	61
France	1959	67
Urban Studies		
United States	1929	51
United States	1945	
Small city		78
Large city		81
France	1948	82
Britain	1950	70
Britain	1951	72
France	1958	67
Britain	1971	77

SOURCE: Ann Oakley, *Woman's Work: The Housewife Past and Present* (New York: Pantheon, 1974), p. 7.

of economic production in the household was also cut off. Thus, women have slowly been forced to become consumers, purchasing items for the daily needs of their families. The economic role of women in the home has been subverted from the active production to the passive consumption of goods and services. As we will see in the next chapter, the potential for job satisfaction and fulfillment from the acts of consumption are far less than from production.

The large number of women employed outside the home today consequently bear the double burden of two jobs, at least one of which has many far from satisfying aspects. Household responsibilities are most often not shared between husband and wife, even if both hold outside jobs. On the average, working women are occupied at least eighty hours per week by their jobs and their homes, while their husbands average about fifty hours of work per week. This is true throughout the industrialized world, as Table 3 shows. The data indicate that in the countries of the Eastern bloc, where it is expected that women work outside the home, they still have the overwhelming preponderance of household duties.

There is a change in the attitude of many young couples who are trying to work out an equitable solution to dividing the responsibilities of homemaking and marketing, cooking and dishwashing, which are no longer considered by them to be the sole domain of women. Once there are children in the family, however, equitable solutions are difficult to sustain, since child raising just does not accommodate a nine-to-five schedule. Because at least one parent must maintain this or a similar schedule to earn a living, the other parent must, and presumably wants to, care for the children, especially very young children. In almost all families, the person who assumes the responsibility for the children is the woman and for the breadwinning, the man.

TABLE 3. SUMMARY OF INTERNATIONAL STUDIES ON
MALE AND FEMALE HOUSEHOLD HOURS

Although in countries like Sweden and the United
States there has been a movement to equalize the burdens
of housework, great inequities still exist. The International
Labor Organization also found that "there is a clear correlation between the time spent on child care and related
activities and the age of the youngest child." (p. 64)

URBAN WORKERS

	Females	Males
Finnish Committee on the Position of Women in Society	4 hours/day	less than 2 hours/day
France, 1966–1967	3.2 hours/day	1.2 hours/day
Japan	3 hours/weekday	less than 1 hour
1972 Leningrad Survey	⅔ of females complained of fatigue, no leisure	

SOURCE: ILO, *Equality of Opportunity and Treatment for Women Workers* (Geneva, 1975).

It is not necessarily true that such role assignments are
taken up by young couples simply because they are the
traditional ones. The practical matter is that men can earn
more money than women can. Another major roadblock to
the division of household responsibilities in families with
children is that housekeeping tasks increase enormously in
time and volume when children are present. Cleaning,
laundry, marketing, and cooking become endless tasks
during the years when children are young.

So while the women of the modern era are in the process
of recovering their lost economic territory, they are doing
so at the same time that society has failed to recognize the
great obligations of the modern home. While the historical
perspective of Myrdal and Klein with regard to the nineteenth-century suffragettes is still true today—

However revolutionary womens demand for the right to
work . . . in fact they were not striving for a new thing but
for the restitution of their lost share in the scheme of

economic affairs. . . . The work had been moved from the home, and the women wanted to move after it, as men had done not so long before.[8]

—the problem is that *all* the work has not been moved. The drudgery of housework and the responsibilities of child and family management were left behind, unrecognized. The modern working woman is on permanent, unpaid overtime.

Mommy Mythologies

Fertility Fictions

Once the current increase in the number of women in the workplace is viewed as part of a movement among women to regain the economic productivity that they had had for centuries, it is worthwhile to examine more closely the popular theories introduced earlier of why women are returning to work in order to see where the theories fall short. As has already been noted, the smaller size of the modern family is a factor often cited for the increasing participation of women in the workplace.

Family-size decline is substantiated by annual birth-rate statistics, which reveal that the number of children being born per 1,000 women of childbearing age—the annual general fertility rate—is currently at a low point. This means that women are, *on the average*, producing fewer children, and hence, the average family size is smaller. However, there are far more women bearing children and raising families now than ever before in this century.

The apparent inconsistency of these statements arises from the statistical methods used to determine population trends. For example, all women of childbearing age—that is, between the ages of 15 and 44 years old—are treated alike in the calculations. Annual general fertility does not take into account the age of the mother or whether her child is her first-born or her seventh offspring. Since the only datum considered is that a live birth has occurred, many unwarranted generalizations about women, their individual rates of reproduction, and their family size are incorrectly drawn from fertility rates.

That the annual general fertility rate does not reflect the childbearing patterns of most women becomes obvious when the fertility of women bearing five or more children is calculated separately from the fertility of the rest of the childbearing females, as shown in Figure 2. Such a calculation shows that from at least 1910 until about 1960, the majority of American women either bore no children or had but one or two children during their lifetimes.

Until the 1950s, about one out of every five women who reached the age range of 35–39 years old had not given birth to any children. About another 20 percent gave birth to only one child. Since the 1960s the percentage of women with no children or one child has dropped drastically to just about one out of every ten women of childbearing age.

Women who gave birth to five or more children throughout the twentieth century represented only a small fraction of the total population. But the children from large families represented a very large fraction of the total births. For example, in 1920, while only 25 percent of the 35–39-year-old female population gave birth to five, six, seven, or more live children, these births represented 56 percent of all the children born to women of that age group. In 1930, 19 percent produced 47 percent of the children. If only the women having seven or more children are considered (see the inset in Figure 2), then 30 percent of the children born in 1920 were mothered by 11 percent of the females.*

Another interesting way to look at this is to consider that almost one out of every three adults whose mother was born between 1881–1885 belonged to a family of seven or more children, but only about one out of every ten

* This figure is actually an underestimate, since it is based on the assumption that the largest family size was seven children. In fact, there were families with eight, nine, ten, or more children, but reliable data are not readily available on the actual numbers. The underestimate is still good enough to illustrate the point.

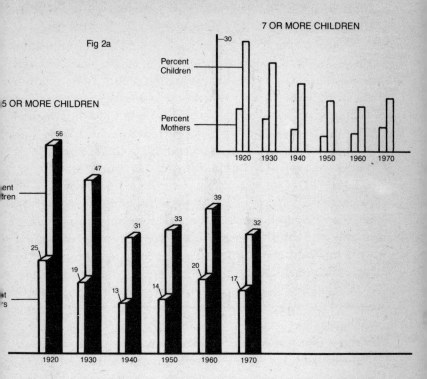

Figure 2. DISTRIBUTION OF WOMEN AND CHILDREN ACCORDING TO
FAMILY SIZE

Figure 2a (above) shows that while a relatively small number of
women gave birth to five or more children, they produced a dis-
proportionately large percentage of the total number of children
born. The inset in 2a shows that women bearing seven or more
children produced an even more disproportionate percentage.

In contrast, Figure 2b (p. 24) shows that the majority of women
gave birth to no, one, or two children and thus were producing a
proportionately smaller percentage of the total number of offspring. The data are calculated for women in the age group
35–39 who gave birth to live-born children.
SOURCE: U.S. Vital Statistics.

families (counting single women as a family) was this large.
If one were to ask each adult of this generation how many
siblings were in his or her family, chances are about one out

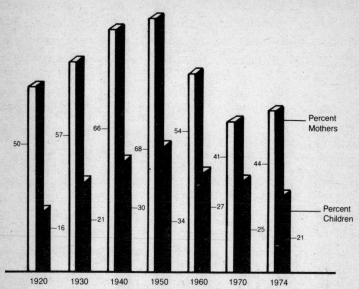

Fig 2b

0, 1, 2 CHILDREN

of three that the answer would be seven or more.[9] It is no wonder that many people associate those earlier times with stories of large families, like *Cheaper by the Dozen*. A good portion of the people around did indeed come from large families, although large families were far from the majority.

The relatively small number of women with large families were reproducing at a rate that at times was almost nine times as great as the majority of women with small (no–two-child) families. The statistical result of a small group of women bearing so many children is that changes in the birth rate of these women will have a disproportionate impact on the total fertility figures for all women. If one woman who would have given birth to seven children gave birth to four children instead, her decreasing birth rate would have the same effect on general fertility figures as three women bearing two children rather than three.

It is the decrease in the size of very large families that is one of the important changes that has occurred during the twentieth century and that has had a strong effect on the birth and fertility rates. The bar graph in Figure 3 tells the story. Both ends of the bar, one end representing big families, the other representing no-children or one-child families, are shrinking, while two-, three-, and four-child families are steadily growing.

This is in contrast to the annual general fertility rate for each year since 1910, as shown in Figure 4, which reveals wide variations during this century. The late 1940s, often called the baby boom years, had record highs in fertility, while the 1970s have been years of record lows. The dip in fertility of the 1930s corresponds to the Great Depression, while the baby boom is generally attributed to the end of the two wars and to an era of economic prosperity. Thus, while fertility may be a good correlate of economic and social conditions, it is a poor one for determining trends of importance to women as individuals. It is certainly an inadequate measure, as we have seen, of the actual number of women participating in childbearing in our society and an invalid measure of their availability for work-force participation.

The Permanent Pregnancy Ploy

Since increased female work-force participation is usually attributed to women completing their families at an earlier age, as well as to the smaller size of families, it is useful to examine birth statistics to determine childbearing patterns with the age of the mother taken into consideration. When this is done, it is seen that about 95 percent of all small families are completed before a woman reaches the age of 35, and about 90 percent of all large families of five or more children are also complete by this time. *This has been true throughout most of the twentieth century.*

The stability and relative youthfulness of the age of family completion over the past decades mean that most women have been free to assume roles other than childbearer for

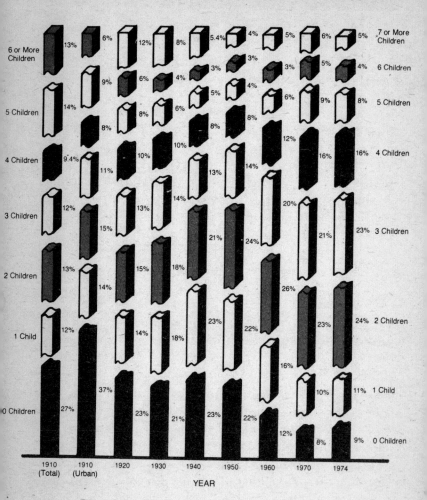

Figure 3. PERCENTAGE OF WOMEN BEARING 0–6 OR MORE
CHILDREN 1910–1974

The bars represent the percentage of women bearing 0, 1, 2, 3, 4, 5, 6, or more children in each of the years shown. Trends have clearly changed from large numbers with 0- and 1-child families to almost universal childbearing.

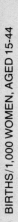
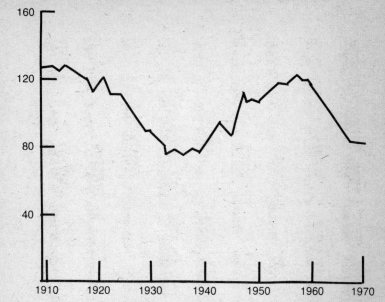

Figure 4. ANNUAL GENERAL FERTILITY, 1909–1970 (FERTILITY RATES PER 1,000 WOMEN AGED 15–44 YEARS)
The fertility rate is the birth rate among women of childbearing age, defined as the total female population between the ages of 15 and 44.
SOURCE: U.S. Vital Statistics.

many years. The age of childbearing cannot possibly explain work-force trends. Further, the sizable number of childless women have always been free from childbearing responsibilities and burdens, a fact generally overlooked.

Breaking down the general fertility rate by age of the mother reveals great differences in birth rate among women of various age groups. The most child-productive years are between the ages of 20 and 24, followed by the 25–29-year-old age group. These are the two age groups with the most rapidly rising birth rates over the years. The relative birth rates since 1917 of various age groups are plotted in Figure 5.

It is especially interesting to note the steady, low birth-rate level over the years of women over 35 years of age.

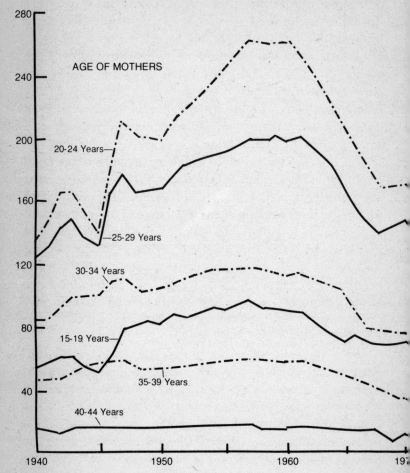

Figure 5. BIRTH RATES BY AGE OF MOTHER, 1940–1970 (LIVE BIRTHS PER 1,000 WOMEN IN EACH AGE GROUP)

The graph illustrates that the birth rate for all women is not the same. The years between 20 and 24, and between 25 and 29 are the most child-productive, while women above the age of 40 have consistently refrained from childbearing.

SOURCE: U.S. Vital Statistics.

During this century these women, though still fertile, have consistently refrained from childbearing. It is also interesting that the fertility of 30–34 year olds has varied very little when compared to the rapid rise of the rate of younger women. The births attributable to this group range from one quarter to one third of the combined birth rates of the 20–29 year olds; so, for purposes of explaining work-force participation, we can even say that many women were free to enter the work-force by the age of 30, further weakening the purported relationship between childbearing-age and work-force-participation rates.

The interpretive problem involving fertility stems from the fact that in calculating general fertility rates, all women are perceived as potential childbearers. This implicitly assumes that all women in the age range of 15–44 years are permanently potentially pregnant. (It is only fair to add that statistics are readily available on the birth rate among women of various age groups. Unfortunately they have not been used in assessing the potential of female work-force participation with respect to the age of childbearing.)

The Maternal Mortality Myth

Along with smaller families and earlier childbearing, another reason which is supposed to account for more women working is that women are living longer. Since at least the turn of the century, the life expectancy of female adults has been long enough to allow the average woman to work until normal retirement age, if she wished. Thus, while there has been an ongoing increase in life expectancy, it can hardly be used as an explanation for the increased number of 35-year-old women in the work force. Rather than explaining increased work-force participation, changes in longevity can be used as a good indication of how many years of retirement the normal woman can expect after age 65.

It is consistent with the apparent need to define women with respect to their childbearing capacity that the sharply reduced rate of maternal mortality (death due to the complications of pregnancy and childbirth) is generally credited with allowing women to live longer and hence be able to work. It is true that maternal mortality, a once major cause of death, has been largely eliminated, and this has contributed to the greater longevity of women; but neither of these facts has any impact on female work-force participation. Again the misunderstanding arises from the uncritical use of statistical data.

In the discussion of life expectancy, it makes a great deal of difference whether one is interested in life expectancy at birth or from adulthood. Life expectancy at birth is based on the death rate, from all causes, of the entire population. The death rates of children and infants will be part of the calculation. When many people die either before 1 year of age or during their childhood, the average age of death for the entire population will be low. If the deaths of the zero through 1 year olds are eliminated, for example, the average age of death will rise sharply. Modern America has, of course, seen a drastic reduction in infant and child mortality, which has resulted in a marked increase in life expectancy at birth.

If one is calculating the life expectancy of people who have already reached adulthood, however, that average will not be affected by infant and child mortality rates, since adults are no longer at risk for these causes of death. The life expectancy of 35-year-old females is based on the death rates of all females 35 years old and above. Life expectancy so calculated will be a much more accurate indicator of changes in the death rate of adults. Trends in female life expectancy at birth and at age 35 are compared in Figure 6.

The Bane of Biological Superiority

The perception of women as the medically and biologically stronger sex is a curious contradiction to the practice of medicine itself. During the last century, phy-

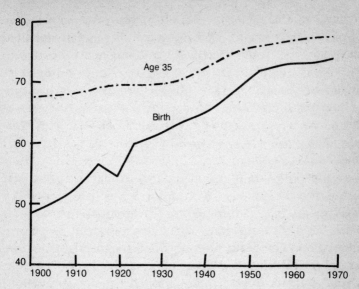

Figure 6. FEMALE LIFE EXPECTANCY AT BIRTH AND AT AGE 35,
1900–1970
Since at least the turn of the century, the life expectancy of the
adult woman has been greater than 65 years. The rising life
expectancy from birth is a reflection of the decline in infant
mortality.
SOURCE: U.S. Vital Statistics.

sicians sought to make invalids out of well women. Menstruation, pregnancy, and childbirth, all normal events, were
treated as illnesses, and women were confined to bed, under
medical treatment. Today, in leading medical texts, menopause is still classified as a disease of the ovaries, although
menopause too is a perfectly normal part of life. Women
are still encouraged to visit physicians regularly and do
indeed visit them more often than do men. They are over-
medicated and overtranquilized. Twenty-nine percent of all
American women used psychotherapeutic drugs in 1973, as
compared with 13 percent of American men. While the
benefits of the annual physical examination for men are
hotly debated in the press today, no one is questioning the
yearly internal examination for women. Thus, while women

are healthier than men, they are treated as sicklier, and normal female functions are unduly subjected to the close scrutiny of medical practitioners. Unfortunately, the scrutiny seems to end when the health of women is impinged upon by their obligations of home and work, or in the study of most major nonfemale diseases.

Not only has the life expectancy of the adult woman been long enough to allow her many years of productive labor, but it is greater than that of the male at every age, from birth to death. Women are healthier, survive more illnesses, and succumb to fewer chronic diseases than men. The superior mortality of women is well summarized thus:

> A biological factor is indicated by the lower death rates among females at every age in industrialized countries; further, there are even fewer female than male stillbirths. The higher life expectancy of females in Catholic teaching orders as compared with males in such orders, when the people in both orders live celibate lives under similar social and environmental conditions, also supports the biological hypothesis . . . females appear to be genetically superior.[10]

Inasmuch as women are less likely to succumb to coronary heart disease, the leading cause of death in America today, they are omitted from major studies on the relationship between environment and lifestyle, and heart disease, even though the differences in statistics between men and women could be scientifically enlightening. It is ironic that the Multiple Risk Factor Intervention Trial (MRFIT), one of the largest, most expensive, and potentially most useful medical experiments ever carried out, excludes women. The program, which initially screened 370,599 men for risk factors in coronary heart disease, is intensively following 12,866 of those deemed to be above average risk. Half of them are also participating in "intervention" clinics designed to help with weight and diet control, and giving up smoking. Although the female diet is virtually identical to that of the male and the rate of women smoking is increasing at alarming proportions, women are nonetheless omitted from these studies because they are stricken with fewer heart attacks before the onset of menopause, when their rate begins to climb.

The MRFIT Annual Report carries a warning against discrimination:

> DISCRIMINATION PROHIBITED: Under provisions of applicable public laws enacted by Congress since 1964, no person in the United States shall, on the ground of race, color, national origin, sex or handicap, be excluded from participation in, be denied the benefits of, or be subjected to discrimination under any program or activity receiving Federal financial assistance. In addition, Executive Order 11141 prohibits discrimination on the basis of age by contractors and subcontractors in the performance of Federal contracts. Therefore, the Multiple Risk Factor Intervention Trial must be operated in compliance with these laws and executive order.

It is difficult to reconcile the theory of nondiscrimination with the practice. It is also difficult to accept that women are being denied the opportunity to participate in the intervention clinics, which are growing more successful each day. The techniques that help women control their weight and their smoking habits may be different from those that help men. We won't know from this program. Furthermore, there is a sharp increase in the rate of heart disease among women after menopause. Female hypertension, or high blood pressure, then exceeds that of males. Surely a productive area for research would be those female hormones that apparently confer on pre-menopausal women some protection against heart disease.

The situation is analogous to Oakley's analysis of the absence of women from sociological studies. She cites that because women are less likely than men to be criminals, they are excluded from criminality studies. Thus, while there is a rising incidence of criminality among women, the trends are not analyzed, and there is no accurate baseline data from which to evaluate trends. The female criminals are ignored, and the differences between men and women are largely unexplored, as are the medical differences just discussed.

The nature of women's work, at home and on the job, is conducive to disease; yet it is almost impossible to draw any conclusions as to whether, in fact, women are developing diseases or shortening their potential life expectancy because of their work, since, in addition to a lack of baseline data, women are usually excluded from investigations in the area of occupational health as well. The exclusions are based on sexual stereotyping and on the inability to recognize the importance of women as workers. For example, in discussing the relationship between Type A aggressive, compulsive behavior and heart disease, the promoters of the Type A behavior theory of disease state:

> Why, you might ask, do most American white women nevertheless appear to possess so much protection against coronary heart disease? Because there are *comparatively* few Type A American white females as completely immersed as males in the contemporary economic and professional milieu that nourishes the development of Type A behavior pattern. Most American women, at least in the immediate past, have remained in their homes, and although they have had many chores to do, relatively few were constrained to work under conditions whose essence consisted of deadlines and competition and hostility. The mother of growing children, of course, does suffer many anxieties, and she at times does have too many tasks to perform, but the effects are clearly less pernicious.[11]

The circularity of the reasoning is obvious. The unfamiliarity with household routine is pathetic. The stereotyping is abominable. And the omission of women from major studies is widespread.

Consider another example. A major monograph on the effects of workplace stress on health, published by the National Institute of Occupational Safety and Health (NIOSH),[12] excluded women workers, although the social sources of stress for women are equal to, if not greater than, those for men. Another NIOSH publication[13] repeatedly cites the classic work of Dr. Anna Baettjer, *Women in Industry*, published in 1946, as one of its most current references on the occupational health status of women workers, although Baettjer herself wrote thirty years ago that she was including the sections on occupational health not so much to present information but rather to point out the great need for investigation in the area. As we will see in the discussion of occupational health, the potential problems are many and varied, yet no massive research is being carried out.

On the one hand, when it is convenient to consider women biologically superior, their superiority is used as an excuse for exclusion from studies on chronic diseases. When it is convenient to regard women as weaker and to stereotype them as homemakers and not as workers, they are then omitted from occupational health studies as well.

The Paradoxes of Legal "Protection"

The contradictions between the biological fitness of women and their treatment as weak or inferior are particularly apparent in the history of protective legislation, where legal constraints on employment have resulted from the definition of woman as perpetual childbearer and as member of an otherwise physically inferior sex. Special labor laws for women have never been a simple issue of owner-employers versus workers, or of government guarantees of good working conditions. They have always been indelibly mixed with basic issues of women's rights and society's general perceptions of the role and limitations of women.

In the 1920s, for example, activist organizations, like the Women's Trade Union League and the Consumer League of New York, staunchly supported protective legislation for women. Other activist groups, like the Women's League for Equal Opportunity, opposed special rules for women. They felt that "restrictions on the conditions of labor should be based upon the nature of the industry, not on the sex of the workers. . . ."[14] They worried that the shorter work-week legislation would "discriminate against women and handicap them in competing with men in earning their livelihood."[15]

Some labor historians see the movement for protective legislation for women as a means of winning rights for men from "behind women's petticoats."[16]

> In order to put an end to evening overtime work the men workers in the textile mills made a long and determined fight for a night work law for women which should prohibit their employment after 6:00 P.M. and thus force the closing of the mills at that hour.[17]

Protective legislation for women has tended to help establish the right to better working conditions for all workers. Up to the turn of the century, workers had very limited legal recourse to do anything about their horrendous working conditions, and even the state could not prescribe minimum standards of employment. For example, in 1905 the United States Supreme Court ruled that the State of New York could not restrict the hours of work in a place of private employment. In that case (*Lochner* v. *New York*) the court held that bakery-worker Lochner's right to make contract under the Fourteenth Amendment had been violated by state legislation prescribing the number of hours a week that a person could be employed. The Court viewed each worker as an individual, under individual contract at work. Such a view of workers is quite conservative and, of course, defeats legal workplace standards, worker organization, and the inherent strength that arises from united ranks. In 1905, seventy-two-hour working weeks and employment of 10-year-old children for twelve-hour days were common practices. Individual contract was meaningless, since workers, in desperation, were willing to work under any conditions available. Individual choice existed only in legal theory.

The fight for protective legislation for women workers provided a break in the doctrine established by the Lochner case. In 1908, in *Muller* v. *Oregon*, the United States Supreme Court held that the State of Oregon could indeed impose a ten-hour-day work limit for women. Opponents of the law had argued that there was no relationship between a shorter work day and public health, safety, and morals; that it was a denial of due process to restrict the working day.

The Court disagreed:

> That woman's physical structure and the performance of maternal functions place her at a disadvantage in the struggle for subsistence is obvious. This is especially true when the burdens of motherhood are upon her. Even when they are not, by abundant testimony of the medical fraternity continuance for a long period of time on her feet at work, repeating this from day to day, tends to injurious effects upon the body, and as healthy mothers are essential to vigourous offspring, the physical well-being of woman becomes an object of public interest and care in order to preserve the strength and vigor of the race. . . . Differentiated by these matters from the other sex, she is properly placed in a class by herself, and legislation designed for her protection may be sustained, even when like legislation is not necessary for men, and could not be sustained. It is impossible to close one's eyes to the fact that she still looks to her brother and depends upon him. Even though all restrictions on political, personal, and contractual rights were taken away, and she stood, so far as statutes are concerned, upon an absolutely equal plane with him, it would still be true that she is so constituted that she will rest upon and look to him for protection;

that her physical structure and a proper discharge of her maternal function—having in view not merely her own health, but the well-being of the race—justify legislation to protect her from the greed as well as the passion of man. The limitations which this statute places upon her contractual powers, upon her right to agree with her employer as to the time she shall labor, are not imposed solely for her benefit, but also largely for the benefit of all.[18]

The regressive doctrines of the Lochner case had been overturned. This new liberal doctrine was a driving wedge, establishing the constitutionality of legislation for the general improvement of all working conditions. Within seven years the ten-hour day was found constitutional for all workers (*Bunting* v. *Oregon* [1917]). But the gain was made on the basis of sexist generalities about the special weaknesses and biological roles of women.

In the 1920s, the conditions in industry continued to be so outrageously poor that only the most benighted observer could fail to see the need for universal change. Despite this need, it is well documented that there was collusion among various organizations and political forces to devise "protective" legislation specifically designed to keep women out of certain areas rather than to improve conditions of employment for all workers.

While many manufacturers and manufacturers' associations sought defeat of all progressive legislation, many of the specialized craft unions were eager to see the passage of protective legislation that would insure that women could not become competitors. According to the Women's Bureau,[19] the active lobbying by the craft unions involved in the skilled trades of grinding and polishing was instrumental in the passage of an 1899 New York State statute prohibiting women from using grinding and polishing machines.

It was not pure male chauvinism that motivated these men. The presence of female labor in a trade or industry inevitably meant the lowering of all wages. That this was all part of a vicious circle seems to have escaped the reasoning of the lobbyists and unionists. As long as women were discriminated against and forced to take whatever jobs they could get, at whatever rate available, they remained an economic threat. Protective legislation in some cases accentuated the economic stress, and the circle was not broken.

Not all labor organizations were opposed to equal rights for women, with several state labor bodies active in the push for such reform. Some of the stronger labor organizations had already gained a shorter work week for their members. Their gains would be consolidated when they were spread throughout industry. It was eventually accepted that the generalities about the weaker sex would make it easier to obtain restrictive laws.

Once the constitutionality of protective legislation was established, and the laws passed by the more advanced states, restrictive laws for the employment of women workers gradually spread throughout much of the United States. It is difficult to assess the actual health effect on women, since the forty-hour work week, minimum wage, and other fair labor standards now apply to both sexes. Legal protection has served as an excuse for not hiring or promoting women in some areas, but it is not clear that the discriminations against women at work would not have continued even without the constraints of the law. Now that most protective legislation has been struck down by federal statute, it will be interesting to see what new patterns emerge: Will the mythologies about women at last be set aside, or will new legal mechanisms be devised to perpetuate the myths? We have seen that the generalizations about women as perennial propagators and members of a "leisured," weaker sex are not true. We are left with no alternative but to consider that there are powerful social and economic factors of a woman's life besides the utilization of her womb.

CHAPTER TWO
WORK, STRESS, AND HEALTH

ALL LIVING THINGS, even plants, respond biochemically to their environment. For example, when a person is exposed to the cold, she will shiver. This is a sign that the body is stimulating heat circulation and also contracting blood vessels at the surface of the body to minimize heat loss. Shivering is part of a specific biological response to a physical stressor, cold. Or suppose that a person is called upon to make a speech before a large audience. Naturally she may feel nervous, her heart may pound, her palms may be sweaty and her face flushed. There may be "butterflies" in her stomach. Again, the body is responding biochemically to its environment. The visible effects are signs of internal activities. This time the stressor is not physical and measurable like cold, but rather emotional, taking the form of stage fright.

Each of these stressors produced a different specific response. Each also set off a virtually identical pattern of biochemical response, called the generalized stress response. Some aspects of the stress response are shown in Figure 7. One result of stress is a temporary rise in blood pressure. Whether the source of the stress is cold, a fever, or the excitement of a football game, a rise in blood pressure

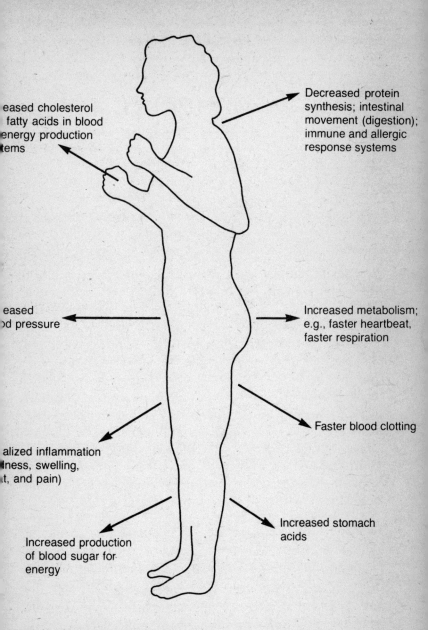

eased cholesterol
fatty acids in blood
energy production
tems

Decreased protein
synthesis; intestinal
movement (digestion);
immune and allergic
response systems

eased
od pressure

Increased metabolism;
e.g., faster heartbeat,
faster respiration

Faster blood clotting

alized inflammation
lness, swelling,
t, and pain)

Increased stomach
acids

Increased production
of blood sugar for
energy

Figure 7. ASPECTS OF THE STRESS RESPONSE

occurs. Because a woman's environment, both at home and at work, has many varied sources of stress, it is of great importance to understand how stress relates to health.

The Stress Response

We can think of the stress response as a mechanism for adapting to the environment. In fact, some scientists call the stress response the general adaptation syndrome. It may not seem plausible that the body responds to different inputs in an identical manner. Indeed, when Dr. Hans Selye, who can be considered the father of modern stress theory, first began presenting his observations on the general adaptation syndrome, or G. A. S., he was greeted with skepticism, disbelief, and sometimes hard and bitter criticism. According to Dr. Selye, the stress alarm system works like a fire alarm system. Notice of a fire can be sent to a fire station by making a phone call, by pulling the handle of a fire alarm box, or by breaking the glass in an electrical alarm unit. All these different inputs cause a bell to go off in the firehouse, setting into motion a preset series of actions that mobilize the firemen.

Dr. Selye parallels this situation to one in which a biological organism will respond to many different inputs with a predetermined set of responses that enable it to meet demanding circumstances. The alarm can be a burned finger, a sick child, a family argument, or a broken leg. It can be a physical condition like cold or noise. Whatever the form, the condition that makes a physical or emotional demand is met with the same stress response.[1]

In an attempt to relate the stress response to what might have been its primitive function, stress is sometimes called a fight-or-flight reaction. Confronted by a physical threat, the body understandably activates its alarm system so that maximum energy is available for meeting and combating an emergency, or for fleeing, if that is the logical alternative—hence the term "fight-or-flight." Calling up energy reserves to meet the stresses of life means wear and tear on the body, since even the best-designed machine has a limited capacity for working. Energy production and wear and tear are major costs of coping with the various aspects —physical, chemical, and emotional—of our environment. Although this sort of energy cost is not exactly measurable in the way that it is possible to determine the amount of gasoline required to drive a mile, its effects can be observed by the increased incidence of disease and disabilities related to stress.

Mechanisms of Stress

As has already been noted, one of the main functions of the stress response is to generate energy to cope with stressors. Another is to insure that all organ systems are operating efficiently in order to use most productively the extra energy available. Virtually every major organ system is involved in stress, hence the origin of the term "generalized stress response." Table 4 summarizes some of the organ changes that occur when a human undergoes a stress response. Although a detailed discussion of the mechanisms of stress is not feasible here, we will briefly examine the biology involved in order to gain some understanding of the relationship between stress and disease.

The Nerves and Glands

Stress mechanisms are controlled by glands and nerves. Glands produce extremely potent chemicals, called hormones, which travel through the bloodstream as messengers used for initiating, halting, or modifying the actions of organs and systems. Most biological functions depend on specific hormones for chemical direction.

The nervous system begins in the brain, the master controller of nervous system function. Major brain pathways

TABLE 4. SELECTED BIOLOGICAL ASPECTS OF THE STRESS RESPONSE

SELECTED EFFECTS ON TARGET ORGANS	SELECTED BIOLOGICAL RESPONSES	SELECTED POTENTIAL ADVERSE EFFECTS
Pituitary and Adrenal Function Stimulated	*Indirect:* (a) Affects all systems listed below *Direct effects:* (b) Increased concentration of cholesterol in blood (c) Increased concentration of blood sugar	Risk factors in heart disease
Blood	Increased clotting time	Risk factor in heart disease
Kidneys	(a) Cell structure can be damaged by adrenal corticoid hormones (b) Secrete pressor substances, which constrict blood vessels and possible decreased excretion ability	(a) Kidney disease can result (b) Can result in hypertension, which in turn is risk factor for kidney and heart disease
Thyroid	Stimulates metabolism in all organs	(a) Increased heartrate—risk factor in heart disease
Fat Tissue	Releases free fatty acids	Risk factor in heart disease
Gastrointestinal Tract (stomach and intestines)	(a) Suppresses movement; changes surface conditions (b) Stimulates gastric acid secretion	(a) Risk factors for duodenal and stomach ulcers, ulcerative colitis (b) Colon cancer (??)
Blood Vessels	Inflammatory changes resulting in constriction	Risk factor in artery disease, heart disease, and kidney disease
White Blood Cells and Lymph Gland	Depression synthesis and function	Decrease immunological response: increased disease susceptibility (??)

extend from the brain down the spinal cord, branching out from the spine and eventually linking up with every muscle, vein, artery, and organ in the body. Electrical impulses, which travel along this vast network of nerves, stimulate the production of hormones directly at the microscopic nerve endings and junctions. They are exactly the same as the hormones produced by the glands, but they don't circulate; rather, their function is to stimulate local muscular and tissue activity.

Nerve endings are, of course, located throughout the body. Major nerves are located in the major organs, and tiny nerves in the smallest parts. There can be no muscular activity without nerve stimulation. Thus, for example, when the spinal cord is severed, the muscles controlled by the nerves in the section of the cord that has been cut off from the brain are paralyzed, will no longer receive stimuli, and will no longer function.

Most of the nervous system is independent of conscious perceptions. Electrical impulses instruct the heart to beat, the lungs to breathe, the stomach to digest, and the muscles to expand or contract, without intellectual input. Lacking such an independent, or autonomic, nervous system, life would perish, for the detailed biological requirements of living would spontaneously outrun the conscious capacity to control muscle and tissue activity.

When stressed, the brain stimulates the pituitary gland, which functions as a sort of central endocrine control because it produces several hormones that stimulate other glandular functions. Specifically, in energy production, the pituitary secretes ACTH, which causes the adrenal glands to secrete several hormones, as shown in Figures 8 and 9. Chief among these is epinephrin (adrenaline), which acts on the muscles and fat tissues, causing them to release various chemicals that have been stored in the tissues as energy reserves. The reserves can be quickly mobilized and converted to blood sugar, or glucose.

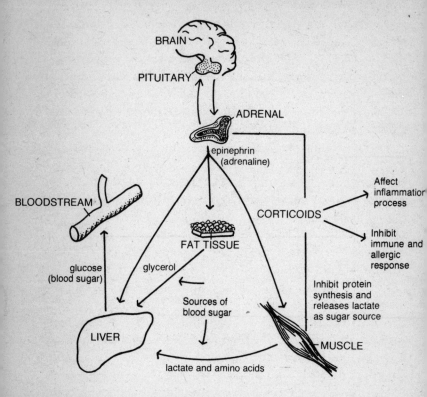

Figure 8. STRESS AND BIOCHEMICAL ENERGY MECHANISMS
Stress mobilizes body reserves for energy production. The response is an increased utilization of normal pathways, as shown.

Energy Production

The stored chemicals travel through the bloodstream to the liver, which acts like a chemical factory, converting them into glucose. Glucose is used directly by the heart and other organs as a source of energy. Adrenaline also stimulates the fat tissue to release free fatty acids—FFA's—which can be oxidized directly by the heart for more energy. The FFA's further suppress the liver's normal process of break-

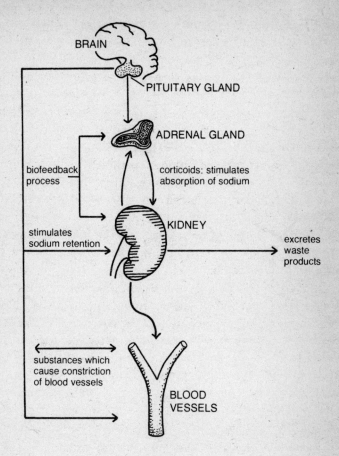

Figure 9. STRESS AND BLOOD PRESSURE
The hormones secreted in response to stress influence sodium retention and kidney function, which regulate blood vessel contraction and hence blood pressure. There is also direct action of the pituitary on the vessels.

ing down glucose, since there is obviously no sense in the liver both synthesizing and breaking down glucose simultaneously.

Hormones called corticoids are produced by the adrenals as well and cause the release of lactate by the muscles. The corticoids have the added function of suppressing the normal protein-building activity of the muscles. When protein synthesis is suppressed, amino acids, which are used as the chemical building blocks of proteins, travel to the liver, where they too can be converted into glucose for additional energy.

Blood Pressure

Blood pressure is related to the stress response via the adrenal glands and the kidneys, as shown in Figure 9. The kidneys help to control blood pressure by regulating the salt concentration in the blood and by secreting substances (pressors) that cause the blood vessels to constrict. Constriction of blood vessels decreases the total volume and raises the blood pressure in much the same way that running water through narrowed pipes raises the water pressure.

The adrenal glands secrete another hormone, aldosterone, that increases blood sodium content, which in turn acts as a signal to the kidneys to secrete pressors. Constriction of the vessels is also stimulated by the pituitary gland.

Elevation of blood pressure is probably related to the need for greater blood flow to accommodate faster respiration and heartbeat, and to the need for circulating blood chemicals more efficiently; but continuous high blood pressure, or hypertension, is a serious disease.

Local Injuries and Stress

Up to now the discussion has dealt with generalized reactions to sources of stress; but if stress is the result of a localized injury, such as a burn or a cut, then a local inflammatory process, as well as a generalized response, will be initiated. The inflammation of local stress is characterized by redness, swelling, heat, and pain. It is a process designed to cope with foreign proteins, like bacteria, and to isolate the affected part. When a local injury takes place, white blood cells rush to the site. These cells surround the proteins, like bacteria, and ingest them. The pus that accompanies inflammation consists of dead white cells and foreign protein, as well as other cellular debris.

Inflammation also consists of hormonally stimulated swelling of tissues, part of a biological attempt to isolate the injured site to keep the injury localized. Tissue cells proliferate and literally barricade the inflamed area. Without this inflammation process, bacteria would freely circulate through the blood and attack vulnerable organs, and even the most minor infection could be fatal.

Like high blood pressure, inflammation itself can be a serious health problem as well as a protective mechanism. For example, if the foreign substance that causes the response is pollen, the characteristic inflammation that results is commonly known as hay fever. Since the pollen represented no threat, the mechanism itself, rather than being protective, has become the disease. Rheumatism is another inflammatory disease. It is not clear what the causative agents or conditions of rheumatism are, but it is the inflammation itself that has the debilitating effect. Acute attacks of this disease can sometimes follow an emotionally or physiologically stressful event.

Anti-inflammatory Agents

In contrast to the inflammation that characterizes the local stress response, the generalized stress response produces hormones (cortisones from the adrenals) that suppress the inflammation. Cortisones are, in fact, often prescribed to alleviate the pain and suffering of inflammatory diseases like arthritis. This anti-inflammatory response is another potential cost of the stress emergency production, because it results in a decrease in the production of white blood cells, an essential part of the body's immune system for fighting infection. Under stressful conditions, therefore, the body will be more susceptible to infectious disease. Many people who suffer from chronic diseases are under constant biological stress and contract infections very easily. For instance, patients with cancer who are hospitalized for treatment are sometimes isolated to prevent contact with infectious disease sources.

The anti-inflammatory reaction may be part of nature's system of balance, which seeks to prevent the pain, swelling, and irritation of local inflammation from becoming more dangerous and debilitating than the original injury itself.

Stress and Ulcers

When the brain responds to stress, it automatically sends a signal to the major nerve in the stomach, which stimulates gastric acid secretion. While the acids in the digestive tract are capable of dissolving tissue, the lining of the stomach and intestines is normally protected from being dissolved in its own fluid. Steroids, which are also released during stress, somehow decrease the ability of the intestinal lining to withstand the stomach acidity. This can lead to ulceration of the lining.

Peptic ulcers are thus another disease that is related to stress. Most people have heard of "executive ulcers," attributed to the stresses of administrative and executive responsibilities. Unfortunately, ulcers are not confined to any one social class, nationality, sex, geographical area, or diet. About 10–12 percent of the world's population is afflicted by the disease.

Shock, major infections, heart attack, cancer, and other severe physiological problems can cause the spontaneous formation of peptic ulcers, most probably as a result of excessive stimulation of the stress response mechanism. There are, of course, other factors related to ulcers, but the emotional and stress aspects play an exceedingly important role in this disease.

Other Biological Costs of Stress

The stress response, with its increased energy production and quickened reaction rates, is not a gratuitous gift of nature. Like all earthly things, it must obey the law of conservation of energy. If, as shown in Figure 8, some energy for the stress response is obtained from chemicals that have been diverted from making proteins, then the body will be deprived of some of the protein it needs. Since protein building is essential to all living things, and since we, as humans, must keep replenishing ourselves, then responding to a stress costs us some protein. Similarly, energy is required to synthesize the hormones so instrumental in regulating the response. This is not "free" and, in fact, can be measured in physical energy units like calories. Calories are obtained from food. Caloric energy that is used for stress is not available for other biological functions. Energy costs are part of the wear and tear of stress.

It is important to realize that the mechanisms illustrated in Figures 8 and 9 are not solely stress response pathways but are normal biochemical pathways activated by many conditions, *including* stress. The stress response is part of the basic life biochemistry. Biochemical reactions are not static but are in a state of balance, fluctuating to meet the demands of the internal and external environments. The stress response is part of the balance; and under usual, or even slightly stressful, conditions, stress will produce only minor fluctuations in the normal biological pathways. When the fluctuations are small, stress, at worst, may use up a little of our "adaptation energy" supply and, at best, may provide us with enough excitement to make being alive worth the trouble.

But if the fluctuations from balance are large or if other disease processes are also present, stress can represent a serious threat to health, perhaps even to life itself. Often stress is part of a vicious circle in which a disease acts as a stressor, producing a stress response, which aggravates the disease, which leads to more stress, and so on.

The fluctuations from steady-state that stress represents are involved in the susceptibility to most diseases; that is, although stress may not cause a disease, it can alter the path the disease takes. Sometimes this is beneficial, as when cancer, following periods of general stress like infection, has gone into remission. On the other hand, cancer is also known to develop at sites of chronic tissue injury and chronic local stress. This is *not* to say that stress can cause or cure cancer but to show that the course of a disease can be affected by it.

Heart Disease and Stress

Heart disease and other diseases of the circulatory system are also related to stress. Like so many chronic diseases, cardiovascular diseases are not caused by a single agent but have been correlated to the factors listed in Table 4. There are several factors common to both heart disease and stress, since stress effects both a rise in blood cholesterol and changes in fatty acid and blood-sugar content.

The various factors involved in causing diseases like heart disease are called risk factors. One way to determine the risk factors of a disease process is to study large populations of people both with and without the disease to see how the two groups resemble each other and how they differ. The presence of a risk factor does not imply that the disease always follows. Although smoking is listed as a risk factor for heart disease in Table 4, there are smokers who do not develop heart disease. Cigarette smokers are statistically more likely to develop the disease and hence are at greater risk. In addition, smoking can only be considered a factor in heart disease, since nonsmokers also develop it. Other factors can include diet, heredity, environment, and lifestyle. A particular risk factor will interact differently with each individual depending on the other risk factors present and on the general makeup of the person and her environmental history.

The greatest risk factor of coronary heart disease is having been previously stricken. Stress plays an important role here. People who are already ill are generally more likely to suffer greater stress effects. Part of the medical regime for caring for an acutely ill coronary patient is to prevent stressful input. Most people know of victims of fatal heart attacks whose final attack was brought on by physical trauma or emotional duress. The effect of stress on an already ill person is, of course, of importance in other diseases as well.

Perhaps the most meaningful way to look at the stress problem is to say that extraordinary or continually unwanted stress costs us energy, deprives us of tranquility, facilitates the occurrence of some diseases, and even outrightly causes others.

Some stress is natural and necessary for life. Other stress, like the death of a loved one, cannot be avoided. The mechanisms are far from understood. Science cannot explain the death of a spouse from natural causes in just a few short weeks after the death of a lifelong marriage partner. The biology of much of life is still far beyond us. It is logical, therefore, to seek to prevent and alleviate sources of stress and disease, and thereby to preserve and extend meaningful and healthy life.

Social Sources of Stress

Researchers have devoted a great deal of effort to identifying social sources of stress and the consequent physiological effects. Unfortunately, few of these studies have included women. This means that although we know a good deal about the stressful effects of job dissastisfaction, job tension, work overload, and responsibility as such, we know rather little about how these parameters affect women.

It is reasonable to assume that the things that make a job dissatisfying and stressful to a man also make it dissatisfying and stressful to a woman. Throughout this discussion we will make that assumption. But it is difficult to estimate how great the effect the added burden of home responsibilities, which has already been discussed, really is.

The direct relationship between stress on the job and disease is complex, but it is clear that job stress and demands can lead to increases in disease risk factors, such as increased cholesterol levels and hypertension. And even if stress does not cause physical ailments and disabilities, it still can lead to mental suffering and ill health, a sufficiently exorbitant price to pay for earning a living.

The human ego needs challenge and pride just as the human body needs nourishment and rest. Failure to obtain such challenge and self-esteem is stressful. Control of one's working conditions is a crucial factor in job satisfaction as are the utilization of one's skills, and adequate financial and social rewards.

Job Dissatisfaction

Job dissatisfaction is a major source of occupational stress and is related to physical aspects of work as well as to one's feelings about work. If a working person is satisfied with her work, then the health effects of job stressors, such as long hours or excessive responsibility, may be lessened. Conversely, interesting work carried out under oppressive conditions can be very dissatisfying. Satisfaction is obviously a composite of many factors. A woman's ability to be satisfied with her work will also be a function of how well she can juxtapose the responsibilities of home and family, if she has them, with her job.

A worker whose skills and abilities are underutilized on the job is likely to be dissatisfied, especially with work that demands constant repetitive motion and/or tasks paced by a machine. Assembly-line work is one clear example of such alienating labor. About 15 percent of working women are employed in factories, many of them in assembly-line jobs. In fact, according to the government task force report *Work in America,* "women are . . . overrepresented on the assembly line—the worst jobs in the economy."[2] Although the number of assembly-line jobs is decreasing each year, the negative characteristics of assembly work, such as rigidly identified and structured tasks, have spread to many other jobs. Keypunch operators, laboratory technicians, typists, coders, and telephone operators are also subject to monotonous, uncreative, rigid tasks, often controlled by a machine. In addition, at least another 25 percent of the female work force is employed in clerical jobs, which also have automaton-like characteristics. Because satisfaction derives from self-esteem and a sense of accomplishment on the job, it will be enhanced by variety, autonomy, and meaningful responsibility, but diminished by boredom, job insecurity, and relative powerlessness.

Another factor in the discontent associated with such employment can be attributed to the requirement of skills far below the qualifications and expectations of most workers. For instance, let us consider the effect of formal education on expectation and preparedness for work. Our society places a great deal of prestige and emphasis on formal education. A person with a college degree is led to expect a rewarding and interesting job. But if the only type of work open to that person is a dull clerical position, then the inability to meet her expectations of an interesting career can be a serious source of stress. This is not to say that both educated and uneducated workers are not bored or that both groups are not equally capable of performing more skillful tasks. Rather, it is a reflection of an additional kind of social burden: unfulfilled expectations.

The discrepancy between high expectations and low social and economic status of jobs was the major factor of female job dissatisfaction cited by an extensive survey on working conditions. Because of the great disparity in job placement between men and women, women were nearly twice as likely as men to be negative about their jobs.[3] It may be even more stressful for an overqualified person to be in a dull job than for a person who, while experiencing the same boredom and dissatisfaction at work, has not been led by society to expect anything better.

It is very difficult to draw firm cause and effect conclusions about women's education, their workplace status, and their expectations, however, because the extensive socialization process, which created the concepts of woman's work, woman's role, and woman's place, is also reflected in the training of women for employment. Other authors have discussed the psychological factors and implications of role fulfillment, so there is no need to discuss them here. Suffice it to say that the vast majority of women students are enrolled in programs that destine them to "women's work" or that give them no vocational skills at all. On the other hand, when women have gained diversified skills and training, they have found it very difficult, if at all possible, to gain prestige and rewards in fields outside the areas of women's work.

OCCUPATIONAL SEGREGATION

The Women's Bureau has recently reported that as of 1973, the top fifty-seven female occupations (with at least 100,000 women in each) covered about 75 percent of all the women at work outside the home.[4] When the Bureau examined the top fifty-seven male occupations, its findings were different. The top ten male occupations employed less than 20 percent of all male workers, and the fifty-seven largest occupations included only 52 percent. This means that occupational opportunities and achievements of men are much more diversified than those of women. The percentage breakdown for broad occupational categories is shown in Figure 10a. Further, the fields in which women concentrate are clearly areas of "women's work." In seventeen (30 percent) of the largest fifty-seven occupations, women comprised 90 percent of the work force. In thirty-one (54 percent), women accounted for more than 75 percent of all employees.

It is not difficult to compile a list of the ten major female occupations. Most readers could probably guess what they are.

secretary	sewer and stitcher
waitress	retail salesperson
registered nurse	typist
elementary school teacher	private household worker
cashier	bookkeeper

The more education a woman has, the more likely she is to be employed, as shown in Table 5. More than twice as

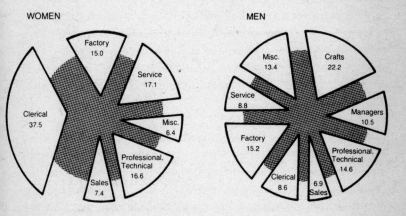

Figure 10a. A COMPARISON OF THE OCCUPATIONAL DISTRIBUTION OF MEN AND WOMEN, 1970

SOURCE: U. S. Bureau of the Census.

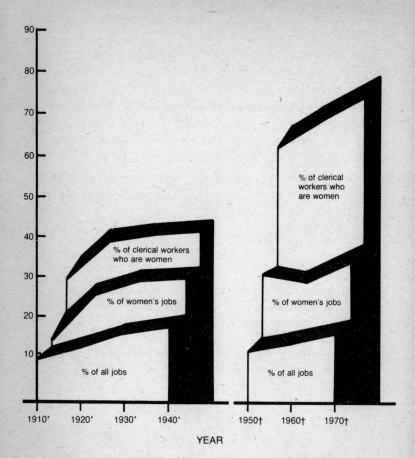

Figure 10b. CLERICAL WORK AND FEMALE EMPOLYMENT,
1910–1970

Although clerical work still represents a small percentage of all jobs (smallest bars), the percentage of female jobs it represents is climbing (middle bars). Further, clerical work is rapidly growing as a female-dominated field (tallest bars). The break in the data arises because census-job classifications were not totally comparable before and after 1940.

* SOURCE: U.S. Bureau of the Census, *16th Census: Population Comparative Statistics for the United States, 1870–1940* (Washington, D.C., 1943).

† SOURCE: U.S. Department of Labor Women's Bureau, *The Economic Role of Women* (Washington, D.C., 1973).

TABLE 5. EDUCATION AND WORK EXPERIENCE

The percentage of women employed in 1975 is given for various educational levels. The table also shows the percent of their adult lives that women with different educational backgrounds were found to have worked in 1967.

LIFETIME WORK EXPERIENCE

	Rate of Employment in 1975	Percent of Adult Life Worked in 1967				
		100%	75–99%	50–74%	1–49%	
Not a High School Graduate	31.6	8.2	16.8	19.5	45.6	9.9	100.0
High School Graduate	52.5	12.1	19.8	20.3	43.3	4.4	100.0
One to Three Years College	53.5 }	20.8	22.6	18.1	36.0	2.5	100.0
Four or More Years College	64.1 }						

SOURCE: U. S. Bureau of the Census, *A Statistical Portrait of Women* (Washington, D.C., 1976).

many women who have completed four or more years of college work than do women who have not graduated from high school. Also, women who have completed education beyond high school have higher work-force participation rates throughout their entire lifetimes.

Further, although men and women workers have achieved almost identical educational backgrounds, the graph in Figure 10b shows that their occupational distribution does not reflect the educational parity. In 1973, one out of every four women on the job was a college graduate and three out of four had a high school diploma; yet, about one out of six female college graduates was still a relatively low-paid clerical worker. The distribution of women in the various occupations by their educational background is given in Table 6. Education has not broken down sexual stereotyping in the workplace.

TABLE 6. EDUCATION AND OCCUPATION

The percentage of women in major occupational groups is given for women with four years of high school and four years of college education, March 1973.

	PERCENT OCCUPATIONAL DISTRIBUTION OF WOMEN	
	High School Graduates	Four Years of College
Professional and Technical Workers	6.3	69.1
Managers and Administrators	5.3	6.2
Sales Workers	76.0	3.2
Clerical Workers	47.0	15.5
Operatives	11.5	1.3
Service Workers[a]	16.6	3.5
	100.0	100.0

[a] Except private households.
SOURCE: U. S. Department of Labor, Bureau of Labor Statistics, *Special Labor Force Bulletin #161* (Washington, D. C., 1973).

Table 7 shows the major categories of female employment. It is first divided into the broad occupational groups used in government statistics, then subdivided into detailed occupations in which female employment exceeded 100,000 in the 1970 census or in which women represented more than 75 percent of the total work force.

Once again, the table shows that most women are clerical workers. In 1973 office work occupied a little more than one third of the entire female work force. Service work, such as waitressing, performing household work, and serving as nurses' aides, and factory work (operatives), such as sewing and stitching, or packing and inspecting on the assembly line, employ about as many women as the professional and technical occupations (e.g., public school teaching and nursing). The percentage is 12–15 percent.

Skilled craft work, such as construction, plumbing, and carpentry—the highest paying of the blue-collar jobs—has never been open to women and still represents a closed-door occupation. Farm work is rapidly dwindling, virtually out of existence, for women as well as for all workers. Many management and professional jobs, such as public administration and architecture, are relatively closed to women as well and represent a job for only one out of every twenty women workers.

Despite the fact that our society is a consumer society, where we must purchase most of the goods and services for our daily lives rather than make them ourselves, sales work represents a shrinking job source for women as well as for men. About 7 percent of all women workers are sales clerks. The absolute number of sales workers keeps climbing, but it does so more slowly than the total number of all new jobs. The same is true for factory work. Blue-collar job opportunities are declining relative to clerical work.

The fact that there is sexual stereotyping does not in itself mean that women's work is dissatisfying. It should be

TABLE 7. WHERE WOMEN WORK

Selected occupations in which women represented 75 percent of the work force *or* which employed at least 100,000 women in 1970 are given in this table.

	# OF WOMEN (IN THOUSANDS)	PERCENT OF TOTAL WORK FORCE	SELECTED (AVERAGE) EARNINGS, 1969 (BASED ON 50/52 WEEK YEAR)		WOMEN'S EARNINGS AS PERCENT OF MEN'S
			Women	*Men*	
Professional and Technical	4397.6	39.9%	$6872	$11,752	58.5%
Accountants	187.0	26.2	6590	11,529	57.2
Librarians	101.5	82.0	6941		
Dieticians	37.8	92.0	5382		
Registered nurses	819.3	97.3	6807		
Health technicians	184.1	69.7	5985	8249	72.6
Social workers	138.9	62.8	7241	8942[a]	81.0
Teachers, prekindergarten and kindergarten	125.1	97.9			
Teachers, elementary	1199.4	83.7	7097	8738	81.2
Teachers, secondary	498.7	49.3	7534	9501	79.3
Teachers, college and university	140.4	28.6	8638	13,126	65.8
Dancers	5.7	81.3			
Managers and Administrators (excluding farm)	1034.3	16.6	6102	11,747	51.9
Restaurants, cafeteria and bar	112.6	34.2	4769	10,463	56.0
Retail trade	100.6	14.6	5859		

Sales Workers	2096.7	38.6	3498	9454	37.0
Demonstrators	36.7	91.1	1857		
Hucksters and peddlers	96.4	78.7	4073	8621	47.2
Salesmen and clerks, retail	1619.4	56.5	5110	7973	64.1
Clerical and Kindred Workers	9910.0	73.6			
Billing clerks	90.5	82.4	4620	5889[b]	84.0
Bank tellers	218.6	86.2	5053	7977	63.3
Bookkeepers	1291.7	82.0	5779	5889[b]	84.0
Cashiers	734.8	83.7			
Library attendants and assistants	101.2	78.6	5240		
Office machine operators	423.1	74.0			
Stenographers, typists, and secretaries	3786.9	96.9	5681, 4936, 5486		
Telephone operators	398.3	94.5	5121		
Craftsmen	524.1	5.0	5277	8730	60.5
Operatives	4222.6	31.5	4334	7493	57.8
Meat wrappers, retail trade	43.0	93.1	4230		
Graders and sorters	30.8	67.5			
Clothing					
Ironers and pressers	146.5	75.2	3386		
Packers and wrappers	332.9	61.9	4460	6386	69.8
Dressmakers, seamstresses (excluding factory)	96.9	95.0	3450		
Laundry and dry-cleaning operatives	261.0	69.8	3386	5603	60.4
Milliners	2.1	89.4			
Textile operatives	247.6	54.8	4379	5595	78.3
Sewers and stitchers	878.7	93.7	3812		

TABLE 7. (Continued)

	# OF WOMEN (IN THOUSANDS)	PERCENT OF TOTAL WORK FORCE	SELECTED (AVERAGE) EARNINGS, 1969 (BASED ON 50/52 WEEK YEAR)		WOMEN'S EARNINGS AS PERCENT OF MEN'S
			Women	Men	
Electrical machinery, equipment, and supplies	113.8	55.2	5006 (?)		
Apparel and other fabricated textile products	74.5	75.5	3723	5440	68.4
Checkers and examiners	355.4	48.5	4897	8407	58.2
Assemblers	519.7	49.5	4887	7493	65.2
Other durable manufacturing (33% in electrical machinery)	134.5	37.6	5006	7769	64.4
Laborers (excluding farm)	294.6	8.4	3960	6135	64.6
Farm Workers	222.3	9.5	2440	3628	67.3
Farm laborers, wage workers	117.7	13.9	2577	3688	69.9
Service Workers	5751.9	60.0	3465	6381[c]	54.3
Chambermaids, maids[e]	202.8	94.8	2823		
Cleaners and charwomen	266.1	56.6			
Janitors and sextons	165.2	12.7			
Cooks[e]	550.5	62.1	3155	5849	53.9
Other food service workers	262.9	74.5			
Counter and fountain	126.3	75.0			
Waiters and waitresses	1002.4	89.0	2796		

Nurses aides, orderlies, and attendants	635.9	84.9	3671		
Practical nurses	233.2	96.4	4919	} 5426	} 90.7
Other health services	847.4	86.2			
Barbers, hairdressers, and cosmetologists	442.4	68.0	3900		
Airline stewardesses	32.2	95.9			
Housekeepers[c]	76.7	71.8			
Housekeepers, private household	761.5	66.0	1482	} 3118	} 64.6
Laundresses, private household	101.5	96.2			
Other private household workers	11.9	94.8			
Child-care workers[c]	131.8	92.8			

[a] Includes recreation workers.
[b] Combines cashiers and bank tellers.
[c] Excludes private households.

SOURCE: U. S. Department of Labor Women's Bureau, *The Economic Role of Women* (Washington, D. C., 1973); U. S. Bureau of the Census, *1970 Census of Population Characteristics of the Population* (Washington, D. C., 1970).

noted, however, that historically the occupational segregation of women has meant that there was an excess supply of female workers, which has driven down wages and exacerbated poor working conditions. Occupational segregation has also meant that there was limited opportunity for advancement and training for women, since there could be no expansion into work roles held by men.

CONTROL OF PACE AND ENVIRONMENT

The more control a worker has over the conditions of her employment and the tasks she must accomplish, the more satisfying the job. For example, a revealing aspect of routine work is found when assemblers on machine-paced work are compared to nonmachine-paced assemblers. Workers whose speed is controlled by a machine are found to suffer from more job dissatisfaction and stress. The difference in strain from machine-controlled speed versus self-regulated speed is a reflection of several things. One is that the regulated work generally tends to be too fast or too slow, and there is no opportunity for altering the pace to relieve the monotony and accommodate personal convenience. But strain can be attributed to the very inability to control this essential part of the work environment.

An interesting sidelight to this study, which involved workers in a Swedish paper mill, was that the workers who suffered the greatest stress effects were not the unskilled workers but the workers whose work required skilled performance on an assembly line. This is, of course, contrary to many commonly held ideas that boredom is worse than anything else. The use of one's skills under alienating, uncontrollable conditions can be more stressful than monotony. Stress can also be induced by jobs where workers must devote some attention and concentration and skill to their work but have no intrinsic interest in it.

Laboratory experiments, both with human subjects and

with test animals, confirm the importance of control over the environment as a stress factor. When a subject is confronted with an experimental stress or challenge and has the option of choosing to end the experiment or escape the challenge, she will not show as great an effect of stress as if she were forced to perform the task for a period of time determined by the experimenter. For example, if a person is performing an arduous task but has been told that she can stop the task when she no longer feels capable of doing it, she will show, on the average, fewer measurable indices of stress. Blood adrenaline levels will be lower than those of the test subjects who perform the same task but without the option to end the experiment; that is, with less control over the situation. Psychological tests confirm this result.

If we apply the concept of control to the jobs that the vast majority of women workers have, we see that most women have no meaningful control over their work environment. Typists, keypunch operators, switchboard workers, and factory operatives are virtually human extensions of the equipment they operate. Service workers, like nurses' aides, waitresses, and cleaning women, are subordinate to the routine nature of their tasks. Sales workers must sell products they do not necessarily like to people whom they must treat as always "right," and answer to the public for a bureaucracy that they cannot control. Sales workers tolerate work areas that are noisy, with no privacy and frequent supervision.

It is very telling to examine professional occupations like social work, library science, elementary school teaching, and nursing—about 15 percent of the female work force. Each of these areas is predominantly populated by women; yet, in each of these fields, the top administrative posts are held by men. For example, a recent survey by John Centra, published by the Educational Testing Service, found that employment opportunities in the private sector are very limited for women with doctorates; and in academia, women are employed in the two- and four-year colleges, while men are hired at the universities. Further, in the university, women are doing the routine teaching, while the men are department heads, academic deans, and presidents, all administrative positions. Being an administrator does not confer ultimate power and control, of course, and being a field worker or subordinate does not necessarily strain and limit a person. However, the disparity between female and male representation in the most prestigious and influential positions does indicate that women are not in control of the direction of their professions. And, of course, the disparity is clearly reflected in the inferior wages of professional women, as shown in Table 8.

Similarly, nursing is almost a totally female occupation; and although nursing administration is a female hierarchy as well, it is made very clear to the nurse and to the nurse administrator, all through training and while on the job, that she "must follow the doctor's orders." Nurses, and indeed all female health professionals, work in a world that is controlled by the male physician and run by the male hospital administrator. There are virtually no professional women workers who exercise autonomy over their working lives.

THE SKILLED OR PROFESSIONAL WOMEN:
ARE THINGS CHANGING?

The major areas in which one can exercise skill and creativity on the job are the skilled crafts and the elite professions. Some experts believe that the 1960s heralded an era of shifts of female employment to such nontraditional areas as carpentry and plumbing, medicine and law.[5] A widely quoted article in the influential *Monthly Labor Review*, in fact, was entitled "Sex Stereotyping: Its Decline in the Skilled Trades."[6] There is little evidence

TABLE 8. RATIO OF EARNINGS OF WOMEN WORKERS TO EARNINGS OF MEN WORKERS, SELECTED YEARS, 1956–1971

OCCUPATIONAL GROUP	ACTUAL RATIOS					ADJUSTED RATIOS[1]	
	1956	1960	1965	1969	1971	1969	1971
Total[2]	63.3	60.7	59.9	58.9	59.5	65.9	66.1
Professional and technical workers	62.4	61.3	65.2	62.2	66.4	67.9	72.4
Teachers, primary and secondary schools	(³)	75.6	79.9	72.4	82.0	(³)	(³)
Managers, officials, and proprietors	59.1	52.9	53.2	53.1	53.0	57.2	56.8
Clerical workers	71.7	67.6	67.2	65.0	62.4	70.0	66.9
Sales workers	41.8	40.9	40.5	40.2	42.1	45.7	47.4
Craftsmen and foremen	(⁴)	(⁴)	56.7	56.7	56.4	60.8	60.2
Operatives	62.1	59.4	56.6	58.7	60.5	65.4	66.6
Service workers excluding private household workers	55.4	57.2	55.4	57.4	58.5	62.5	63.2

[1] Adjusted for differences in average full-time hours worked since full-time hours for women are typically less than full-time hours for men.
[2] Total includes occupational groups not shown separately.
[3] Not available.
[4] Base too small to be statistically significant.

NOTE: Data relate to civilian workers who are employed full-time, year-round. Data for 1956 include salaried workers only, while data for later years include both salaried and self-employed workers.
SOURCE: U. S. Department of Labor Women's Bureau, *Economic Role of Women* (Washington, D. C., 1973).

that this decline is occurring. Most of the change seems to be the result of small, statistically insignificant shifts in employment numbers and a misreading of the meaning of relative rates.

Much of the problem in the interpretation of employment trends stems from the use of relative rates. For example, it has been stated that the rate of increase of women working in the industrial crafts was eight times that of men. That is true, but it is also a rather meaningless marker. Let us take an extreme but illustrative example. Suppose that there were two women employed as craft workers in 1960, but in 1970 that number had increased to twenty. That means that there were ten times as many women craft workers employed in 1970 as there were in 1960. Further, let us assume that the men's employment figures went from eight million to nine million in the same period of time. That would be only a 12 percent increase compared to the 1000 percent increase in the number of women. The increase of eighteen women workers compared to one million males is obviously not indicative of any decline in stereotyping; but if we merely looked at the rates of increase —1000 percent compared to 12 percent—these eighteen jobs would seem very meaningful indeed.

Statistics will lie unless they are correctly calculated and interpreted. If we look at our example in another way, the error of the statistical method is apparent. Between 1960 and 1970 there were one million and eighteen new jobs in the crafts. Of these jobs, .0018 percent went to women and 99.82 percent went to men. The real rate of change must be measured relative to the total number of jobs.

Re-evaluating the statistics in the crafts, we see that between 1960 and 1970 about 765,000 new craft jobs were created. The percentage of all craft jobs held by women increased from 3.1 percent to 5.0 percent. At the same time the female work force in all fields expanded much faster than the male work force. This was to be expected, since the vast majority of males were already employed, while only a minority of working-age women were previously in the work force. There was much more room for female expansion. In fact, for every man entering the work force, there were about two women who did.

If there truly was a decline in stereotyping in skilled craft hiring, then we should expect to see two women hired in new craft jobs for every new man that was hired. What actually happened was that out of the 765,000 new jobs, about 547,000 went to men and 218,000 went to women, or for every two women hired there were five men hired. This is five times worse than nondiscriminatory hiring practices would require.

The figures cited are uncorrected for job attrition and other market factors, so that they overemphasize the positive. If we look at the fields that women entered within the skilled crafts, the situation is even gloomier. Of the 218,000 new jobs created, about 10 percent were in areas like bookbinding and window dressing, which have always been fields open to women. Another 22,000 jobs were in the area of printing and typesetting, which is rapidly becoming obsolete because of technological advances. The Department of Labor's *Occupational Outlook Handbook* cites this area as a poor employment prospect, where the only jobs that can be expected will be those arising from the retirement and attrition of the present workers. There was a decline in male employment in these areas.

By refining the calculations to account for this obsolescence and for the expansion of already female-dominated areas, the hiring ratio becomes six men for every two women, as compared to two women for every man, which is necessary for nondiscrimination. And this discussion has not even touched upon affirmative action programs. Such programs are designed to seek out groups that have suffered discrimination in past hiring practices and to provide them with greater employment opportunities. We can see that affirmative action, which has been touted as a reason for this "decline in sex stereotyping," has had no impact on female professional or skilled craft employment.

Other Sources of Stress

There are other sources of job stress besides job dissatisfaction. Work overload, responsibilities, and deadlines can also be stressful. For example, in one extremely interesting study of public accountants, it was found that the blood cholesterol levels rose and fell with the rising and falling of the seasonal tax work load. Accountants are naturally under a great deal of pressure, both mental and physical, at tax time. They work very long hours, under an obvious and ominous deadline. January 15 is another tax deadline for many businesses as well, so that the weeks preceding this date also represent a stress period.

Researchers who worked with the accountants in the study asked them to keep a detailed record of their work and home activities, as well as of their diets. Blood samples were taken and analyzed for serum cholesterol and for clotting time. The results, some of which are given in Figure 11, show that cholesterol levels followed the variations of job stress experienced by these men. (As discussed earlier in the chapter, cholesterol is a strong risk factor in coronary disease; clotting time is related to the occurrence of strokes.) One conclusion that can be drawn is that the kind of stress experienced by these accountants, and its consequent physiological effects, can, in fact, be related to problems like heart disease, a result that has been confirmed by other investigations.

In this example, job stress consisted of a very long work week, of a strong sense of time urgency and deadlines, and of dealing with clients who were also under stress and pressure. The responsibilities were great, and there was limited ability to control the situation, since deadlines and rules are strictly set by the tax laws.

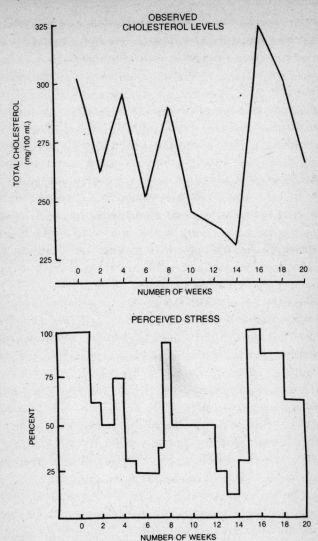

Figure 11. CHOLESTEROL AND STRESS: AN EXPERIMENTAL RESULT
One accountant in the study cited developed his own rating system for his perceived stress (b), which is in good agreement with the serum cholesterol results determined clinically (a).*

* SOURCE: Meyer Friedman et al., "Changes in the Serum Cholesterol and Blood Clotting Time in Men Subjected to Cyclical Variation of Occupational Stress," *Circulation* XVII (May 1953): 852–61.

When responsibilities involve the welfare and supervision of human beings, then the stress is even greater. Woman's role traditionally has been that of caretaker for the needs and well-being of others. She is mother, nurse, teacher, cook, and comforter at home; and she is nurse, teacher, waitress, "gal Friday," and social worker on the job. In fact, the occupational categories in Tables 6 and 7 show that the majority of women workers bear responsibility for others on the job.

Responsibility is a greater strain when workers are given little discretion in dealing with others. For example, clerks and social workers at an unemployment office work with people who are out of work and seeking new jobs and unemployment insurance benefits. Unemployed people are not in the best frame of mind to begin with; and when they must tackle the endless lines, waits, and paperwork of the benefit process, their patience wears very thin. There is frequent verbal violence, sometimes even physical violence; and the social worker and clerk are too often the recipients of this abuse.[7]

Not only is the job at such a center monotonous and uncreative, but sometimes it is also dangerous. Stress arises because of the necessary interactions with an alienated public, in a situation where the worker has no discretionary powers over the rules and regulations set by the state.

At a series of occupational health and safety conferences held across the United States by the American Federation of State, County and Municipal Employees (AFSCME) Union in 1976 and 1977, a major complaint voiced over and over was the difficulty and stress of dealing with the public in just such trying circumstances at various social service centers. In general, it was felt that having the role of the powerless representative of a large and very often unresponsive bureaucracy is a difficult assignment.

Furthermore, public-sector employees complained that

they did not have the typical company-worker relationship of a private enterprise employee. Government workers' salaries are derived from the public coffer. Each benefit they receive is generally perceived as an additional drain on the community's resources. This adds to the stress of the job because seeking improved wages and conditions, especially during times of fiscal crises, is considered almost unpatriotic. In some cases the burden for the fiscal problems of municipalities and states is placed squarely on the workers' shoulders. Yet public-sector workers have the same emotional and financial needs as other workers, and many times they are paid substantially less.

A similar situation applies to health-care workers, since their employer is often a "nonprofit" institution or the government. When health-care workers are faced with working conditions or job requirements that do not allow them to perform as efficiently as possible, they suffer the added burden of knowing that their inefficiency can directly affect the health of a human being. Administrative rules and regulations not in the best interests of the patients, or a lack of facilities and staff preventing them from giving patients optimum care constitutes an even greater source of stress. Health-care workers must also deal regularly with sickness and death, and there are major studies currently under way that are seeking to establish just how great a demand this is on workers' health.

Stress and Job Rewards

The last aspect of social stress on the job that will be discussed is the relationship between stress and psychological and monetary rewards for work. Human beings need to work. They work to attain a sense of fulfillment, achievement, and identity, and to provide themselves with food, clothing, and other necessities of life. In our society monetary rewards are a sign of special value. Getting paid a high salary is a source of pride and achievement for some people. Other people derive rewards from performing meaningful and useful tasks.

Social scientists try to separate these rewards into two categories. They consider pay and prestige "extrinsic" rewards and satisfaction and pride "intrinsic" rewards. Some studies have shown that there is a higher incidence of coronary disease among workers who work for extrinsic rewards. Unfortunately, this has led some prominent researchers to urge people not to seek extrinsic rewards in their work but rather to work for the joy of it.

The trouble with this point of view is the fact that in 1973 more than 65 percent of American workers earned less than $14,000, an amount that is now just about sufficient to support, very modestly, an urban family of four. Most people do not have the option of earning less so that they can get more enjoyment out of their work, because there are not many jobs available that allow a person to use talent and creativity and earn a decent wage. The usual combination that presents itself to workers is one of insufficient extrinsic and intrinsic rewards.

It is difficult to assess quantitatively the relationship between rewards and stress, as there are so many subjective aspects. But rather than setting up sanctimonious prescriptions for leading a fulfilling, less stressful life by shunning the pursuit of wealth and power, let us acknowledge that it is probably very stressful to work arduously and still not have enough money to live reasonably well. Insufficient financial reward is an obvious source of stress and dissatisfaction.

Also, if one works very hard and is rewarded less than someone else who works very hard at the same job, then this too is a source of stress. As we shall see, many women, although hard-working, are underpaid, generally are unable to support themselves or their families, and earn less than men performing the same tasks.

SEX AND WAGES

Although the educational attainment of the two sexes is comparable in each of the employment areas, women earn less than two thirds of male wages in each group. As the graph in Figure 12 indicates, this gap has been widening steadily despite the rhetoric about the changing status of the new working women. Working women suffer the double discrimination of being relegated to women's work roles and of being paid lower wages. Data on average earnings for 1969 for broad occupational groups, such as clerical workers or service workers, are given in Table 9.

The table also shows the earnings as a function of education. Women with college degrees make less than men with

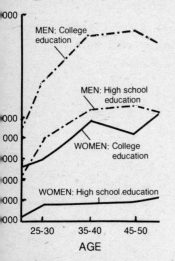

Figure 12a. THE GAP IN WOMEN'S INCOME: A COMPARISON OF EARNINGS FOR MALE AND FEMALE EDUCATIONAL LEVELS

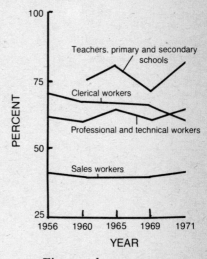

Figure 12b. THE GAP IN WOMEN'S INCOME: AS A PERCENT OF MEN'S IN SELECTED OCCUPATIONS, 1956–1971

SOURCE: Carolyn Jacobson, *The American Federationist* (Washington, D. C., AFL-CIO, July 1974).

TABLE 9. EDUCATION, OCCUPATION, AND EARNINGS

The average earnings of women in occupational groups are given for high school and college graduates. These are compared to each other, and the earnings of female college graduates are compared to male high school and college graduates, March 1973.

	AVERAGE EARNINGS		COMPARATIVE PERCENTAGES		
	Women 4 Years High School	Women 4 Years College	Women 4 Years College to Women 4 Years High School	Women 4 Years College to Men College	High School
Professional and Technical Workers	7819	9232	118	63.9	77.2
Managers and Administrators	6581	10350	157	59.9	86.7
Sales Workers and Clerical Workers	5876	6934	118	53.9	70.6
Operatives	5386	5833	108	54.2	58.5
Service Workers[a]	4551	6278	138	58.4	71.9

a Except private households.
SOURCE: U. S. Department of Labor, Bureau of Labor Statistics, *Special Labor Force Bulletin #161* (Washington, D. C., 1973).

high school degrees in every occupational category, and about half of the wages of equally educated college males. Comparative earning figures for males and females for a few detailed occupations are also shown in Table 9, but these figures are not complete. This is because most of the earnings data in the 1970 U. S. census were not useful for comparing male earnings to female earnings. The occupational overlap between the sexes is not great enough; that is, in most of the detailed occupations for which earnings data were compiled for women, there were no comparable statistics for men and vice versa, a result of sexual occupational segregation.

Women's earnings are a reflection of the social status of their work roles. Women's work is very literally valued less than men's. Jobs that relate to caring for children, for people, for homes, are the lowest on the pay scale. There is far less status in teaching young children than graduate youth. Rewards like pay, prestige, and a sense of achievement are based on how society values one's contribution. Women's work just does not rate very high.

The Stress of Work in the Home

Housework, the "other" job of most working women, shares many of the worst characteristics of dissatisfying paid employment. In an extensive sociological study of housework, Ann Oakley found that the majority of women complained about the drudgery and monotony, as well as the endless repetitiveness, of many household chores. A major factor in their dissatisfaction with housework was that it has no defined beginning and end, so that it is difficult to feel a sense of "accomplishment"—which we have already noted is vital to job satisfaction—especially if children are present, rapidly *un*doing all the housework that has been done.

Many women in the survey, however, enjoyed both the

sense of "being their own boss" and the opportunity to raise children. However, it was almost universally apparent that raising children was considered a separate task from housekeeping and, in fact, that children made housekeeping more difficult. In addition to increasing the amount of housekeeping, children also prevent a person from having unbroken periods of time to spend on housework.

Rewards and recognition are another component of satisfying work. Housework is unpaid labor. Its economic value is not even counted into the gross national product. If a person must purchase the services of cooking, cleaning, shopping, and child care, which the average woman performs in the home, it would cost at least $10,000.

The direct relationship between stress and disease is complex; but it is clear that job stress and demands, especially when juxtaposed with family responsibilities, can lead to increases in disease risk factors, such as increased cholesterol levels and hypertension. And even if stress does not cause physical ailments and disabilities, it still can lead to mental suffering and ill health, a sufficiently exorbitant price to pay for earning a living.

The human ego needs challenge and pride just as the human body needs nourishment and rest; failure to obtain such challenge and self-esteem is stressful. Control of one's working conditions, as well as relief from the burdens of the dual role of work and home, are crucial factors in job satisfaction, as are the utilization of one's skills, and financial and social rewards.

CHAPTER THREE

HEALTH HAZARDS ON THE JOB

THE PHYSICAL ASPECTS of work, like the social ones, can directly affect a working woman's health. While most people associate occupational diseases and industrial accidents with arduous and obviously dangerous "man's" work like coal mining and ditch digging, large numbers of women also work at jobs that present many serious, though often less dramatic, health hazards.

Unfortunately, just as calculations of the nation's fertility assume all women to be potential childbearers, so too is a woman's health on the job usually discussed solely in terms of reproductive capacity. Such a discussion took place at the first major scientific conference devoted to the subject of the occupational health of women workers. Although the fact that the meeting took place was a great step toward the recognition of women as workers, the entire first day was spent on the "risks of toxic substances on future generations" and "birth defects, cancer, and miscarriages" arising from occupational exposures; a large part of the second day dealt with reproductive dangers associated with lead and other job hazards; and the conference ended with half of the last half-day focusing on legal and medical issues related to pregnancy. Other aspects of occupational health hazards were virtually ignored.[1]

Some aspects which remain to be considered are the excessive lifting, bending, carrying, and standing found in the health professions, or the poorly designed work areas, inadequate lighting, and uncomfortable chairs encountered in many clerical positions, which can have adverse effects on workers' health. Sometimes the hazards are physical agents, such as the noise and vibration in a textile mill or the radiation in nuclear medicine or X-ray specialties. Extremes of temperature, dampness, or drafts, which occur in occupations like supermarket meat wrapping and laundry work, are other forms of environmental hazards. Of course, toxic substances, such as chemicals, dusts, and fumes endemic to many factories where women work, as well as to service, cleaning, and health professions, can enter the body and affect internal functioning, and can damage the skin, directly causing skin disease. Bacteria, viruses, and other infectious agents pose an added threat to women when they come into contact with contaminated laundry or dishes, in service work, or perhaps in the laboratory while analyzing biological specimens. Women who work with sick people will be exposed to their disease; similarly, women who work with children and the public sector are also at greater risk of infectious disease.

Furthermore, it is interesting that some of the major health hazards for women at work complement and exacerbate hazards at home. Back injuries and backaches are common to workers on the job as well as to the mother of young children and to the housekeeper at home. Skin irritation and disease are widespread among hospital workers, service workers, and industrial workers just as they are among women in the home role of "chief cook and bottle-washer." Women who care for children at home are also exposed to the many infectious illnesses that young people contract. And, of course, fatigue from long hours of housework and responsibilities is endemic to the dual role of homemaker and worker.

Identifying Occupational Diseases

The true incidence of occupational diseases, for men or women, is not known. Unless the nature of an occupational disease is striking and acute, it will probably go unrecognized or its cause may not be associated with the workplace conditions that brought it on. For example, if a worker in a dry-cleaning plant became sickened, nauseated, and possibly even developed chemical inflammation of the liver (hepatitis) after accidental and massive exposure to a cleaning solvent, her illness could be readily attributed to her job, because she developed a rapid, *acute,* recognizable response to a work hazard. But if the same woman developed *chronic* symptoms of nausea or fatigue from some disorder of her liver that developed after many years of exposure to small amounts of solvent, chances are that her illness would not be correlated to her job, even though work-place conditions may indeed have caused, or at least contributed to, it.

The slow, sometimes even imperceptible, development of chronic disease accustoms many people to their symptoms, such as fatigue or a daily cough. Furthermore, because chronic diseases, unlike rapidly developing and progressing acute diseases, extend over time, their cause may not be readily recognizable. Also, many different conditions or substances may lead to the same chronic effect. The risk factors of heart disease, discussed previously, are an example of multiple causation.

In the example cited above, both alcohol and dry-cleaning solvents could have led to the liver disease, so that a work-induced liver disorder may be either misdiagnosed or actually the result of the combination of chemical insults. When many causes can lead to the same effect, it is difficult to know if any particular cause did; and since most physicians are not aware of the hazards of work, they will generally be overlooked as factors in disease.

The possibility of multiple causes, the vague nature of some of the symptoms, and the length of time chronic diseases take to develop make the scientific aspects of investigating chronic occupational diseases complex. Complexity should not obscure the fact, however, that a major reason so little is known about the effects of occupational health hazards is that so little total effort is expended to study and prevent them. As we have already noted, research on women in this area is especially needed.

Where Have All the Women Gone?

In a massive study of all the occupational health literature published in the United States and abroad, Vilma Hunt found that "literature . . . describing the health experience of women workers is sparse, despite their concentration in a relatively few industries. . . ." She also noted that "it is surprising" how many study designs excluded women.[2] The inability to recognize women as workers and to see them beyond their potential childbearing and homemaking roles is thus quite apparent.

An interesting historical example of this inability, or refusal, on the part of many researchers to recognize that women are a continuing segment of the work force is found in the Women's Bureau Bulletin *Women Workers in Expanding Wartime Industries,* published in 1943.

> The increasing diversity of women's work in the war program has implications not only for greater opportunity to use talents and to secure better wages than in more customary women's employment, it also brings about the exposure of women to toxic materials to which they rarely have been exposed in modern American industry.[3]

Yet in 1928, almost a generation earlier, the Consumers' League of Massachusetts surveyed the extent of female exposure to occupational poisons and tabulated its findings, most of which showed that very early in the twentieth century significant numbers of women were exposed to the same materials and worked in the same industries as those that existed during World War II. The Consumers' League Survey was reported in a major Women's Bureau Bulletin on *Occupational Disease,* a bulletin in the same series as the 1943 publication; however, the wartime reporter apparently knew nothing of the original bulletin. (Figure 13 reproduces excerpts from the two bulletins.[4])

Figure 13. SOME EARLY CONDITIONS OF WOMEN INDUSTRIAL WORKERS

1929 Consumers' League of Massachusetts survey of 55 factories: some types of industrial poisoning

Establishment number	Number of women employees	Poisonous substances
		LEATHER INDUSTRY
1	30	Amyl acetate, butyl acetate, and benzol.
2	5	Do.
4	50	Butyl acetate, denatured alcohol, fusel oil.
7	100	Pyroxylen or nitrocellulose, amyl acetate, butyl acetate, benzol.
9	57	Denatured alcohol.
10	64	Amyl acetate in cement.
11	82	Benzol and wood alcohol. (Doping done by men, but women work near oven room where patent leather is baked and get some of the fumes.)
13	5	Benzol, amyl acetate, and butyl acetate.
14	8	Amyl acetate and wood alcohol. (Doping done by men in adjoining room, but women get some of fumes.)
		SHOE INDUSTRY, INCLUDING CUT STOCK AND FINDINGS
1	100	Wood alcohol, ether, naphtha rubber cement, repairing dope.
2	18	Naphtha rubber cement and repairing dope.
3	190	Methyl (wood) alcohol, patent leather repairing dope, naphtha rubber cement.
4	300	Methyl (wood) alcohol, patent leather repairing dope, ether, shellac, naphtha rubber cement.
5	30	Methyl (wood) alcohol, naphtha rubber cement, ammonia cement.
6	100	Naphtha rubber cement, ether, carbon disulphide for cleaning shoes.
8	300	Methyl (wood) alcohol, acetone, naphtha rubber cement, ether, amyl acetate and butyl acetate in cements.
9	125–150	Naphtha rubber cement, repairing dope.
10	350	Patent leather repairing dope, naphtha, rubber cement, benzol rubber cement.
		RUBBER INDUSTRY
1	800	Carbon tetrachloride, naphtha rubber cement.
2	100	Naphtha rubber cement, sulphur chloride, sulphur.
3	1	Naphtha rubber cement.

6	35	Naphtha rubber cement used by men in small, poorly ventilated room from which women get fumes.
10	3200	Naphtha rubber cement.
11	4	Naphtha rubber cement used by men in small, poorly ventilated room from which women get fumes.
12	200	Benzol rubber cement, carbon tetrachloride, sulphur chloride, carbon disulphide.
15	1	Naphtha rubber cement used by men in small, poorly ventilated room from which women get fumes.
16	2	Do.
17	1	Do.

1943 Women's Bureau evaluation of women's potential exposures to harmful materials during the wartime years

Skin irritants:

Benzol (see also under systemic)	Glass silk
Tetryl	
Mercury fulminate	Materials used in manufacture of plastics
Mica dust	Dyes of various kinds
Pyranol	Cutting oils and compounds

Systemic poisoning:

Lead oxides	Tetryl
Benzol	Mercury
Radium	Carbon monoxide

Respiratory diseases: Silica dust; steel dust; mica dust.
Acid burns—Nitric acid
X-ray burns—X-ray
Heat prostration—Excessive heat

SOURCE: U. S. Department of Labor Women's Bureau, *State Reporting of Occupational Disease: 1934*, Women's Bureau Bulletin no. 114 (Washington, D. C., 1943); U. S. Department of Labor Women's Bureau, *Women Workers in Wartime Industries*, Women's Bureau Bulletin no. 197 (Washington, D. C., 1943).

The conditions of the war years were not new—only the recognition lent to them and to the fact that women shared with men the burden of exposure to toxic workplace conditions. Unfortunately, women still face many of the same occupational health hazards in industry today. These can have a direct bearing on the public at large because much of woman's work involves the public and caring for its needs.

Occupational Health and Women's Occupations

Women, more so than men, are particularly adapted to manual dexterity, assembly lines, use of small drills and punch presses, mailing and filing, preparation of foods, or weaving

—A. W. DIDDLE, M. D.
Journal of Occupational Medicine, 1970[5]

Sexual stereotyping has led to occupational segregation of women. Thus, because so many women do work that is very similar, even in different occupations, they have many hazards in common. Therefore, when the same hazard, like lifting or standing, is encountered in several occupations, it will be discussed at length only once, and the reader will be referred to that discussion when the hazard presents itself again. There are several summary tables and a glossary of occupational health hazards as well.

The Health of Health-care Workers

> She always carried to the sickbed a round, yellow tin box. In it she kept moldly bread, each scrap of bread being added when it was no longer usable for table. The dust from opening the box was a cloud of green. When she dressed a wound she made poultices from this bread and warm milk or water. . . . This she applied directly to the wound and the healing was rapid and clean. She never lost a timber-related patient.
>
> Elizabeth Stone was using penicillin to treat victims of timber accidents in Peshtigo, Wisconsin, 70 years before Dr. Alexander Fleming "discovered" it. . . . Elizabeth Stone cared for the sick as long as she lived. . . . Unfortunately she was less successful with her own health than she was with others.[6]

Before the advent of "modern medicine," it was women like Elizabeth Stone who cared for the sick; today, in the age of technology, it is still the women who care for the sick—but not as highly paid professionals. And just like Elizabeth Stone, today's health-care workers rarely receive adequate health care.

Slightly over half of the more than three million women in health-related work are service workers—nurses' aides, cooks, food handlers, and janitors—as the graph in Figure 14 indicates. One out of five women in health is a registered nurse, and one out of ten is involved in the clerical aspects

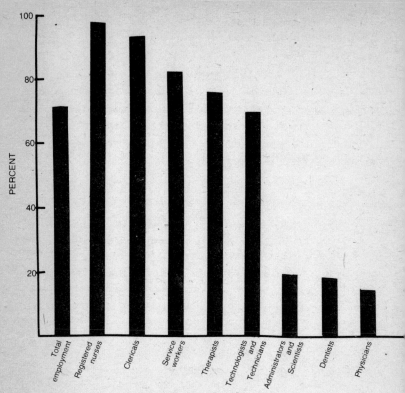

Figure 14. THE OCCUPATIONAL DISTRIBUTION OF WOMEN IN
HEALTH CARE, 1970

SOURCE: U. S. Bureau of the Census.

of health care. Fewer than two out of every one hundred
female health workers is a physician, dentist, administrator,
or scientist.

Most of the women in health care must lift, feed, and
clean up after patients; they work in the least glamorous,
lowest paid service jobs, which are probably the most
hazardous as well. Table 10 shows some of the hazards in
service and other areas of health care. It is immediately
apparent that hospitals and other health-care settings are
rather unhealthy places to work. If you've ever wondered
how people can manage to work with the sick and always

TABLE 10. HAZARDS OF HEALTH CARE

Hospital workers, dentist and physician office workers, laboratory workers, and others are subject to the health hazards categorized below.

HAZARD	SOURCES, EFFECTS, AND PRECAUTIONS
Infections	
	Although many hospitals and other facilities take precautions to isolate infected patients, there will still be contact with undiagnosed cases. In many instances, routine handling of potentially infectious objects and patients may be inadequate.
Viral hepatitis (serum hepatitis)	This serious disease is especially prevalent in kidney dialysis units. Dentists and dental technicians also have an increased incidence, as do clinical laboratory workers and those in contact with drug abusers. Wearing protective gloves during blood taking is a good precaution. Blood specimens should be isolated and disposed of separately if there is any possibility of hepatitis. Kidney patients should be tested for hepatitis B antigen and isolated if result is positive.
Tuberculosis	Widespread in inner-city and other impoverished areas, thus contact with infected patients is possible. When a TB case is diagnosed, those in contact must be kept under medical surveillance and treated if necessary. Routine TB testing of probable cases is advisable. Monkeys are used in laboratories, and are TB carriers.
Herpes simplex virus	Usually comes from contact with infected sputum, especially tracheotomy patients. Protective gloves should be worn, especially if mechanical devices for sputum removal are in use. Service workers should be protected and warned of potentially infected objects. Causes painful skin lesions.
Rubella virus (German measles)	Potential problem in pediatric wards. All females of childbearing capacity should be immunized because of potential birth defects from infection during pregnancy.

TABLE 10. (*Continued*)

Enteric gram-negative bacilli and other fecal contaminants	Germs carried in the feces can be sources of polio and typhoid, for example. Soiled linens and stool specimens should be handled without skin contact. Workers should be immunized.
Staphylococcus aureus	Infections by this organism are endemic to hospitals. Has been found even to contaminate water in patients' flower vases. Care, caution, and cleanliness are essential to minimize risk.

Chemical Hazards

Ozone	Used as a disinfectant and is also produced by office copying machines and therapy equipment with mercury lamps. Extremely irritating to lungs. Ventilation should be provided. Also thought to be similar to X-rays in biological effect.
Anesthetic gases —cyclopropane —divinyl ether —ethyl chloride —ethyl ether —trifluoroethyl ether —ethylene	Have been implicated in causing spontaneous abortions in exposed workers and also possibly birth defects. Exposure occurs in operating rooms, dentist and physician offices, and veterinary and animal labs. Can affect reflexes and possibly increase risk of accidents. Scrubber units must be used with these gases.
Inorganic acids and alkalis	Strongly irritating to the nose and upper respiratory passages, as well as to the skin.
Xylene	Can irritate and crack the skin, and can be absorbed through the body. Although it is used as a less toxic substitute for benzene, it may also have effects on the blood.
Chlorinated hydrocarbons	Used in dry cleaning. Toxic to liver. Many found to cause cancer in animals. Adequate ventilation must be provided.

Hydrogen sulfide	Irritating, and in very high concentrations, can lead to respiratory failure. Long-term exposure may cause chronic lung disease.
Metallic mercury	Used in clinical laboratories, often handled carelessly. Droplets vaporize and can lead to poisoning, which affects nervous system and kidneys. All mercury must be cleaned up.
Phenolic compounds	Easily absorbed through the skin, and very irritating to it. Some compounds are extremely toxic and should not be used. See Bibliography for further references.

Physical Hazards—

Microwave radiation	Sources are microwave ovens (food handlers), diathermy machines (therapists). Can be harmful to eyes and cause cataracts. A controversy exists as to negative effects at very low levels. Should be avoided when wearing pacemaker, or with metal implants.
Lasers	Used in some surgical procedures and laboratories. Avoid all eye contact with rays. Can cause cataracts or other permanent damage.
Ionizing radiation: X-rays, radiochemicals	Can cause burns, birth defects, cancer, etc. Effects are thought to be cumulative. All unnecessary exposure should be avoided. Proper shielding for X-rays essential. Radiochemicals should be properly labeled and disposed of. Monitoring of exposure necessary.
Noise and vibration	Service workers and laundry workers particularly exposed. Can harm hearing ability and is a source of physiological stress. Circulation can be affected by vibration. Hearing conservation and noise reduction programs necessary.
Ultraviolet light	Used in some sterilizing procedures. Can sensitize skin toward chemicals and can burn skin. Can also lead to cataracts. Skin and eye contact should be avoided.
Heat and thermal stress	Laundry and service workers particularly exposed. Adequate breaktime necessary. Can affect heart and circulation. A physical stressor. Engineering control of heat sources should be used wherever possible.

TABLE 10. (*Continued*)

Skin Disorders

Nail infections (onychomosis)

Dishwashers, nurses' aides, and others who must keep hands wet for prolonged periods are potential victims. Protective gloves and other precautions necessary (see pages 125–26).

Allergic (contact) dermatitis

Food handlers, those handling and applying medications and other sensitizing substances are vulnerable. Can cause inflammation and sores similar to poison ivy.

Dermatitis from irritation

Soaps, bleaches, and detergents, as well as phenolics and other disinfectants are irritants. Maintenance workers using oils and solvents also exposed. Can result in cracking and reddening of skin or can lead to sores and infections.

Safety Hazards

Back injuries

Occur from excessive lifting and/or carrying. See pages 94–97 and Table 12 for discussion.

Puncture wounds, cuts

Improper facilities for disposal of syringes and poorly enforced regulations. Can lead to infections. People who administer shots, as well as laundry and service workers, are susceptible. Sharp instruments also a problem.

Abrasions and injuries from falls

Wet floors and crowded spaces full of mechanical devices lead to a high injury rate.

Electric shocks

Many pieces of hospital equipment, especially portable devices, are not properly grounded or insulated. Regular maintenance and safety surveys are essential.

stay healthy themselves, the answer is that they can't. It is useful to examine the problem areas systematically.

INFECTION

An obvious risk in dealing with sick patients is infection. Although most hospitals and other health-care facilities have special precautionary measures for handling patients with serious infectious diseases like tuberculosis and viral hepatitis, there will be many hours of exposure to the undiagnosed cases of such diseases before routine laboratory tests are returned. In addition, direct patient contact is only one of the many ways that health personnel can contract disease.

Handling, analyzing, and disposing of biological specimens, such as blood samples, is a prime method of disease transfer. Hospital surveys have shown that many hospitals are not equipped with isolation facilities for handling the analyses of such dangerous samples as tuberculosis smears. After samples are analyzed they must be disposed of, which means there is potential exposure among the janitorial workers, as well as the people taking the samples, transporting them to the laboratories, or analyzing them. While there are adequate methods for isolation and disposal of dangerous specimens, these methods often are not stringently followed, as the high incidence of infection among hospital personnel shows.

Of course, the possibility of infection is not limited to biological samples. The workers in one blood fractionation facility that has been studied were found to develop hepatitis at the rate of four per hundred each year, a risk many times greater than that of the general population. Furthermore, an even larger number of workers are carrying the infection without clinical signs of the disease themselves. Dentists, workers in kidney dialysis centers, and people in contact with drug abusers are other groups vulnerable to hepatitis infection. Also, many infections other than hepatitis are also spread within health institutions. For example, nurses who come into contact with infected sputum, especially from neurosurgery patients, may develop very painful viral infections on their hands (*Herpes whitlock*) that take some time to heal. The true number and variety of hospital-induced infections among staff and patients are not known. Some are given in the table.

BACK INJURIES

Since many patients are too ill to be self-sufficient, they must be lifted when their beds are changed or when they are transported around the hospital. Lifting heavy patients is one source of back injuries, which are among the major recognized hospital hazards. Despite the high incidence of back problems, however, little has been done to ease the lifting and carrying burden of health-care workers. Hospital beds are not designed for easy lifting, and certainly hospital staffs are far too small to allow cooperative worker efforts which would ease the burdens on individuals. There are other hospital chores that also require lifting, such as carrying heavy cleanup buckets, and lifting and carrying equipment packs. These tasks too could be eased by mechanical carrying devices and better job design.

Back Construction

The back is made up of the spinal column, which consists of twenty-four blocks of spongy bones, called vertebrae. The function of the back is to support the body's weight. Between each vertebra is a cushion called a disc. Strong elastic ligaments surround and bind the bones and discs together, while muscles allow the trunk to move. At least two muscles are required for every movement. Front and back muscles control forward and backward motion, side muscles control sideways bending. A detail of the back structure is shown in Figure 15.

Many people blame their backaches on slipped discs,

which is the condition that occurs when the cushiony disc pops out of its bony framework. Although some backaches are caused by disc slippage, the majority of back problems are really due to strains and injuries to the ligaments and muscles that support the bones. If a great deal of force is applied to the ligaments, such as from lifting an object that is too heavy, the ligament fibers can tear. This is extremely painful and can make the muscles stiff and cramped. When

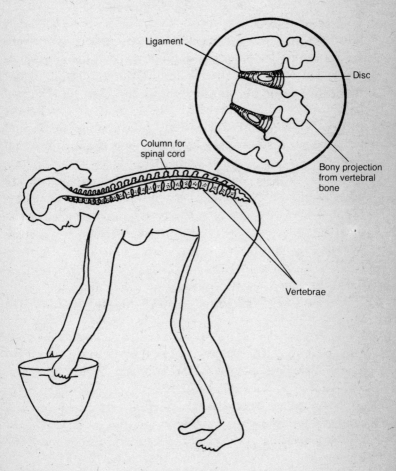

Figure 15. THE BACK

the ligament heals, it will leave a scar. Scarred tissue is weaker than normal tissue, so that the healed ligament is easier to injure again if another force is applied to it.

Because of the increased susceptibility to back injury of the person who has already suffered one, *it is very important to keep the first injury from occurring*. Occupational back injuries can be prevented by restricting lifting and carrying, and by providing chairs, tables, and work areas designed for health. A well-designed area will conform to the body's natural motions and will support the frame of the body. A motion is unnatural if it is uncomfortable to do. "What feels good is good" is probably the best test of a work situation. Table 11 shows the recommended maximum weights that should be lifted by men and women of different age groups. It is immediately apparent that even the smallest and lightest adult patient will be many times heavier than the maximum recommended weight that should be lifted.

If the ligaments are repeatedly injured, they become loosened, so that the discs and joints are not held firmly enough, thereby increasing the chance of disc and joint injury. Injured joints develop bony spurs, which can be observed in an X-ray. This painful, sometimes disabling condition is known as osteoarthritis, or degenerative arthritis. Each joint that is damaged increases the stress on other joints, so that back injuries can progress along the spine. Again, prevention of initial injury is the best cure. If the

TABLE 11. RECOMMENDED WEIGHTS FOR LOADS FOR
OCCASIONAL LIFTING BY UNTRAINED WORKERS

AGE	MEN	WOMEN
16–18	44 lb.	26 lb.
18–20	51 lb.	30 lb.
20–35	55 lb.	33 lb.
35–50	46 lb.	28 lb.
over 50	35 lb.	22 lb.

motion that triggered the first injury can be pinpointed, it should be scrupulously avoided.

When the back muscles are strong and well exercised, they can support the ligaments most effectively. A well-planned exercise program can help maintain good muscle strength. But aging weakens muscles, and lifting heavy patients is too great a load even for a young, healthy worker. Mechanical devices and better-designed hospital equipment are solutions to the back injury problem.

Fatigue can also affect the body's ability to cope with stress and injury, as we have already discussed. The woman worker is greatly fatigued by the dual demands of home and work, by the stress of her job, and by the nature of her work. Improvements in occupational health will obviously require more than mechanical lifting devices.

OTHER INJURIES

Puncture wounds from needles, lacerations from knives and blades, bumps, abrasions, and other injuries also occur frequently in a health-care setting. A large hospital will have hundreds of these injuries among the staff each year. Wounds are particularly dangerous in the hospital setting because of the risk of infection, discussed earlier. Some of the most common injuries found in hospitals and typical occurrence rates are given in Table 12.

A technological revolution is not necessary for eliminating these hazards. Convenient and enforced disposal routines among all levels of personnel, mechanization, and a large enough maintenance staff to handle the work load safely can probably eradicate most injuries.

CHEMICAL HAZARDS

Anesthetics

Exposure to anesthetics among operating-room personnel is an example of how an occupational health hazard may have a direct effect on patient health. Chemicals used as

TABLE 12. TYPICAL HOSPITAL ACCIDENTS AND INJURIES

Selected accidents and injuries encountered in major departments are given. Rates of accidents, which were found in a survey of a large major hospital, are also given. Strains and sprains from lifting and carrying, as well as cuts (lacerations), are the most common accidents.

| | | RATE | |
DEPARTMENT	TYPICAL ACCIDENTS	Total Injuries/ 100 Workers	Lost-Time Accidents/ 100 Workers
Food Service			
Butchers and cooks	Cuts from sharp equipment; infected wounds from bone splinters	14	3.3
Cooks, dishwashers, assistants	Burns		
Food porters	Sprains, back injuries from lifting heavy trays and cases of food		2.5
Nursing Service	Cuts, puncture wounds from syringes, contusions from slipping on spills, strains from lifting patients and heavy equipment	22.1	
Housekeeping			
Laundry workers	Burns from sterilizing and presser equipment; fractures and bruises from extractors, washers and dryers without safety switches; puncture wounds and cuts from needles, blades, etc., improperly disposed in laundry; sprains and strains from lifting	30.3	2.9
Laboratory workers	Cuts and puncture wounds from improperly disposed syringes, pipettes, etc., or from sharp equipment	12.4	0.3

anesthetics have the ability to affect nerve function and can lead to unconsciousness, which is, of course, the property that makes them useful in medicine. But it is also the property that makes them potentially dangerous. Test subjects who were exposed to concentrations of anesthetics normally found in operating rooms were observed to have markedly reduced reaction times and sensory abilities. This raises serious questions about the reaction time of the operating staff during surgery, when their ability to react may be a matter of life or death. Is anesthetic air pollution limiting the ability of surgical staff? We don't yet know.

Many anesthetics can also cause liver damage, although this is generally not a problem for the patient who receives anesthetic treatment for a surgical procedure. However, if a patient or hospital worker does have a history of liver disease, exposure to anesthetics may be harmful.

Anesthetics can also affect the ability to bear children. Operating-room personnel have between two and four times the number of spontaneous abortions that unexposed women do. There are also more birth defects among their offspring than among the unexposed population. There is some evidence that the reproductive capacities of males are also affected. (These hazards and other reproductive hazards of work are discussed in the next chapter.) The National Institute of Occupational Safety and Health (NIOSH) estimates that about 214,000 medical and dental workers are exposed to these gases.

Despite the inherent toxicity of anesthetics, despite the effects on reflexes and responses, and despite the potential for reproductive effects, fewer than 25 percent of all operating rooms are equipped to prevent anesthetics from polluting the air. Dental operating facilities are even more poorly protected. The equipment that can keep the anesthetics out of the air is inexpensive, especially in comparison to the usual cost of medical apparatus, and easy to use, yet there is resistance among professionals and administrators to its installation. While the debate about the effects of anesthetics is being waged in the pages of the professional journals, women workers and other operating-room inhabitants are still being needlessly exposed to anesthetic pollution.[7]

Ozone

Ozone, a chemical form of oxygen, is very effective for sterilizing rooms, but is also very reactive and irritating to the eyes, nose, and throat. Even in concentrations as small as one five-hundredth part of ozone per million parts of air, ozone can severely damage the lungs. In addition, there is evidence that ozone is related to cancer. There really should be no exposure to it.

Since ozone is a gas, when it is generated for sterilizing rooms, it must be carefully contained and controlled. Its use in hospitals is probably not controlled well enough, exposing patients and personnel to needless hazard. (Office workers also have potential exposure to ozone when they use electronic stenciling machines. See Table 14.) Suitable substitutes should be found and ozone used only in emergency situations.

IONIZING RADIATION

Radiation from X-rays and from exposure to radioisotopes is another occupational health hazard of hospitals. Again, health-care recipients, as well as health-care workers, may be at risk. There are about one quarter of a million X-ray units in use in the United States, many of them improperly maintained and emitting excessive radiation.

Ionizing radiation from medical and dental X-rays can have powerful biological effects. (In large doses it can cause radiation sickness, be fatal, or lead to cancer, especially leukemia. Its genetic and reproductive effects are discussed with other reproductive hazards in the next chapter.) But it does not take large doses of radiation to have biological effects. Somehow the effects of radiation are cumulative; that is, many small doses over a period of time will add up. It is not clear whether the total effect of the small doses is less than, equal to, or greater than an equivalent large dose; but in any case, it is very significant to health. That is why exposure standards for radiation are calculated on the basis of lifetime exposures. The cumulative effects of radiation are, of course, important to hospital workers, who may be exposed to only a small amount of radiation at a time.

Despite the biological costs of radiation, X-rays can still be a useful diagnostic tool. For many people the benefits to be derived through its use are worth the small risk involved. (One should not assume, however, that all prescribed X-rays are necessary, or that the machines used are well maintained. The alert medical consumer will ask questions and get other opinions when in doubt.) And, of course, there is *no* health benefit for the hospital worker exposed to radiation while X-raying patients. The only benefit that the X-ray technicians derive is their livelihood, so that any exposure to X-rays is both unnecessary and potentially harmful to them.

There are shielding methods available for blocking X-rays; but for some X-ray techniques, the technician is not adequately shielded and must be near the patient, thereby exposing herself to radiation. Portable X-ray machines are an example. These machines emit a great deal more radiation than the nonportable variety and endanger not only the technician but the patient, other patients, and staff in the vicinity. Table 13 shows the X-ray dosages that are emitted by various diagnostic procedures. Adequate estimates of technician exposure levels are not readily available.

Another source of ionizing radiation in the hospital is radioisotopes, which are used for diagnosis and treatment. Radioisotopes are radioactive forms of chemical elements. Certain elements tend to concentrate in particular organs

TABLE 13. LEVELS OF RADIATION EMITTED FROM TYPICAL X-RAY PROCEDURES

X-RAYS: TO PATIENT	SKIN EX-POSURE (MR)†	% REC. STAND‡	AVERAGE BONE MARROW DOSE (MRAD)†	MODIFIED % RECOM-MENDED STANDARD*
Chest X-ray (side view)	132	1.3	10	5.9
Barium enema (side)	6220	62.2	231	136.0
(front)	1030	10.3	109	64.0
(rear)	1030	10.3	115	68.0
IVP [injected dye, kidney view] (front)	885		79	
				89.0
(side)	1170	20.6	72	
GI series (4 views)	5479	54.8	287	168.0
Dental (front teeth)	1110		2.9	3.0
		22.8		
(back teeth)	1170		2.8	

RADIATION: TO SURROUNDINGS

Cobalt 60 chemotherapy			150–170 mrad/hr will
Dental: low voltage	0.05–0.1 (per cycle))		vary depending on
high voltage	0.15–0.22 (per cycle)		contact time and
			distance

† mR = milliroentgens.
 mrad = one thousandth of a rad; a unit of radiation dosage. A rad is approximately equal to a rem.
‡ Recommended standards = 10 roentgen/year.
* This is a percentage based on a recommended standard of 0.17 rem/year. The standard is supposed to exclude medical X-ray. The percentages in this column have been supplied for comparison purposes only, not for evaluating over-exposure.

the way iodine concentrates in the thyroid, so that levels of radiation emitted from various parts of the body can tell a diagnostician many things about a person's health—and expose workers to radiation at the same time. The tendency to concentrate in particular organs also makes radio-isotope therapy useful in cancer treatment. Levels of radiation emitted by radio-treated patients are also given in the table.

Office and Clerical Work

Office workers are not generally thought to be subject to health hazards on the job, especially when their work is compared to such dangerous work as coal mining and construction. Yet, there are potential health problems for office employees that should not be ignored simply because they are not immediately fatal or overwhelmingly hazardous. We have, in fact, already encountered some of the hazards in the discussion of social sources of stress and the dual role of homemaker and worker; and Table 14 outlines some of the physical hazards endemic to clerical occupations.

SITTING, POSTURE, AND HEALTH

Many clerical jobs involve long hours of sitting at a desk, writing, keypunch operating, answering telephones, typing, or performing similar tasks. Sitting for unbroken lengths of time can be uncomfortable in the short run and detrimental in the long run, particularly if the chair and table are not properly designed.

A chair must allow a person to sit with a minimum amount of pressure on the thighs, which are soft and easily compressed; otherwise, blood circulation can be blocked, resulting in pooling in the lower part of the body. This pooling causes the veins to dilate and can lead to, or aggravate, hemorrhoids, the very uncomfortable dilation and swelling of the veins at the opening of the anus. Blood pooling is also a complicating factor in varicose veins (see pages 118–19) and other circulatory problems.

A chair seat that is horizontal or shaky can cause back muscles to stiffen. Unless a chair is constructed so that the back muscles are in an optimum position, the lower back will also gradually stiffen and possibly begin to ache. The most relaxing position is when a person is leaning slightly forward, as shown in Figure 16. Another good position is sitting up straight with the lower back area supported by the backrest of a chair.

TABLE 14. HAZARDS OF OFFICE AND CLERICAL WORK

The exact nature and extent of office hazards are not known. They will, of course, vary from office to office. While office work is far less hazardous than many other kinds of work, there still is no reason for any health risk to be present. The control of adverse office conditions can usually be readily accomplished.

HAZARD	SOURCES AND EXPLANATIONS
Excessive sitting	Improperly designed chairs can lead to backache; can aggravate hemorrhoids, varicose veins, and other conditions relating to the circulation of blood.
Fatigue, muscular and mental	Boredom as well as intense concentration can be fatiguing. Eyestrain from insufficient illumination or glare as well as muscle strain can also contribute.
Noise	Noise can be annoying and/or harmful. High levels, like those of keypunches and computers, can adversely affect hearing, while low levels may be stressful and interfere with communication.
Muscle strain	"Writer's cramp" from overexertion of small hand muscles may arise. Typists and keypunch operators may strain tendons of wrist (tenosynovitis).
AIR CONTAMINANTS	
Ozone	Many copying machines and some switchboards may generate this toxic gas, which is a form of oxygen. Characterized by a sweetish smell, it can lead to irritation of eyes, nose, and throat. Exposure should be minimized, and exhaust vents installed near machines.
Spores, dusts, and asbestos	Rarely, insulation in air shafts may become exposed, leading to the spread of cancer-causing asbestos. This should be immediately eliminated. Improperly cleaned and maintained air conditioners can harbor and spread spores, which can produce allergic responses in susceptible individuals.
Benzene and toluene	These contaminants are found in rubber cement and some "cleaners." Contents should be checked. Benzene is associated with various blood diseases, and toluene can cause a drunken state, which increases the risk of accidents.
Methanol and ammonia	Used in many duplicating-machine solvents, these substances can be very irritating to the eyes, nose, and throat.
Organic solvents	May be found in various stencil machines, "erasing" compounds, and other office products. Contents should be checked and can be identified for toxicity by reference to books listed in the Bibliography.

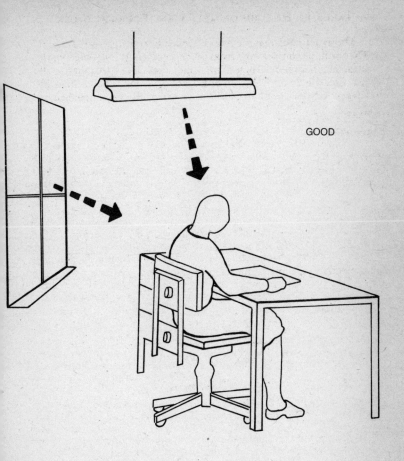

GOOD

Figure 16. SEATING AND LIGHTING DESIGN
To avoid glare, neither natural nor artificial light sources should be directly in front of the desk. Chairs should match desk height and be adjustable, supporting the lower back and sloping slightly forward.

Jobs that require a great deal of concentration will cause a person to tighten all her muscles gradually and subconsciously. If, while doing a demanding job, you have found your face set in a frown or your jaw set tight, you have experienced involuntary muscle tightening in response to

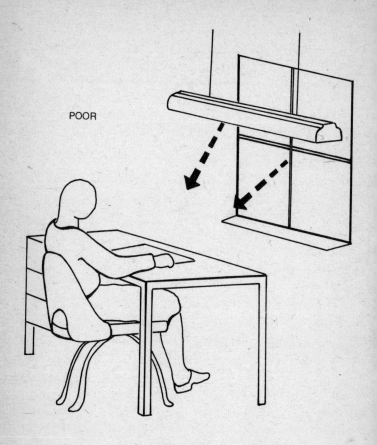

Figure 16b

stressful input. Such muscle tightening makes unnecessary muscular energy demand, causing muscles to become fatigued and painful. Similarly, straining some muscles by sitting incorrectly can lead to whole body fatigue. Of course, the design and height of tables must complement the design of chairs.

Many office personnel like file clerks must spend a good part of the day standing, which puts a stress on the circulatory system, on the muscles, and on the back, legs, and feet. The effects of standing are discussed more fully on pages 118–21.

WRITING

It is not only the large and long muscles that are fatigued from the requirements of work; the muscles of the hands, fingers, and wrists can also suffer from overexertion. It is thought that when a muscle is used at more than 50 percent of its capacity, it begins to fatigue. Not all the muscles are the same size, as Figure 17 shows. The small muscles of the fingers and hand that are used for writing, sewing, or other precise motion are fatigued rather easily because they are so small and delicate; as a result, it will not take extreme demands to exceed the 50 percent capacity. When the muscles are fatigued, they become painful, a condition sometimes called writer's cramp.

If the tendons of the wrist, which connect the muscles to the bones in the wrist, are overexerted or stressed, they can become inflamed. This is called tenosynovitis and sometimes afflicts typists and other office workers whose work makes excessive demands on these tendons.

LIGHTING, EYES, AND OFFICE WORK

Proper illumination is necessary in order to work efficiently without undue strain, and different tasks require different illumination levels. Reading or transcribing from poor paper, especially if the writing is in pencil, requires more light than reading inked material on high quality paper. Similarly, filing all day will require more light than will occasional filing. Working with ledgers and figures demands the most intense illumination.

Lighting should be adequate for the task but should not produce a glare. If the light source is not positioned properly with respect to the work that is being done, it may reflect

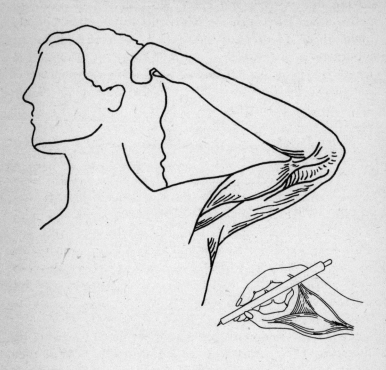

Figure 17. SMALL AND LARGE MUSCLES
The comparatively small muscles of the hand and wrists are fatigued more readily than the long muscles, which can be developed to relatively great strength and capacity.

off the work surface into a working person's eyes. Lights that are too bright can cause visual fatigue as well. There are standards for lighting levels, which are available; and if a woman wants to see how the lighting in her office rates, light levels can easily be assessed with the standard light meter used in photography.[8] Figure 16 also shows some principles of proper lighting.

Fluorescent fixtures—the kind generally found in offices—

should never be placed immediately in front of a desk but on the side instead, and every effort should be made to position desks between rows of lights rather than directly under them. Fluorescent lights emit ultraviolet radiation; but there is no evidence, positive or negative, about the health effects of this. Of course, natural light and windows are an excellent source of illumination, but many of the office workers of today seem destined to spend their days in the center of large, windowless rooms.

Modern technology has produced another potential hazard to the eyes: television-like display screens, or CRT's, used for computer input and output. A woman who works with a display throughout the day will be watching a flickering screen that has highly contrasting areas of dark and light. The writing is small, and the great contrast between the dark screen and the background light in the room makes the use of CRT's very hard on the eyes, possibly leading to pain and discomfort. CRT's are currently available for interchanging dark and light backgrounds, but this is probably not the total solution.

Some CRT manufacturers warn that people wearing bifocals should not work with a CRT routinely because they will have to strain their necks in order to read the information on the screen. And, of course, one can expect the typical muscle aches and pains that come from sitting for prolonged periods, which we have already discussed.

In the study of (wo)man-machine interactions, it is a well-known theory that work which requires a great deal of attention but which is of little intrinsic interest is very fatiguing. It will certainly be an unusual person who finds the mass of data stored and displayed on the CRT screen of intrinsic interest, so that CRT work will ultimately be quite tiring. Visual fatigue is defined as general weariness arising from the physical exertion of seeing, meaning that more than the eyes are affected.

NOISE

Office workers, as well as many other workers, are exposed to noise on the job. Most office situations do not involve the extreme noise exposure found in heavy industry. The surroundings, however, are noisy enough to be annoying and to interfere with a person's ability to communicate, to concentrate, and to work efficiently. Such noise can be a significant source of stress, similar in its effects to the other sources of stress discussed in the previous chapter. And if noise is loud enough and exposure to it long enough, it can also cause permanent damage to one's hearing ability.

Noise is often defined as unwanted sound, which reflects the fact that it can be annoying and stressful. Annoyance from noise, in turn, is technically defined as perceived noisiness. Because annoyance involves one's perceptions, psychological factors are involved. However, despite this, annoyance can be quantified. Scientists investigating the annoyance aspects of noise have found rather remarkable agreement among different people tested and a good consistency in annoyance test responses in the same subject tested repeatedly.

This consistency among tests and test subjects may be because the annoying effects of noise vary as a function of the frequency and duration of the sound; and since frequency and duration are real, measurable aspects of noise, they apparently outweigh individual perceptual differences in importance. Another factor that affects annoyance is the location of the noise. People generally require a perceived noise level (PNL) at home that is one fourth of the perceived noise they can comfortably tolerate outdoors.

Perceived noise is not the same as loudness. It will be much more annoying if, like a high whistle, sound is concentrated in a narrow frequency range than if it covers a broad range of frequencies, like a bass drum, even though the broad-spectrum drum sound may be perceived as "louder."

Through extensive surveys and tests, experts in this field have developed criteria and formulae for evaluating noisiness. By measuring the frequency distribution, and the intensity and duration of noise, one can calculate the PNL and other measures of annoyance. These measurements have been carried out for a number of environments, such as offices, homes, hospitals, libraries, and churches, as well as for various appliances and utilities. Some of these figures, and data showing the maximum PNL for efficiency and comfort, are given in Table 15.

Examining the data in Tables 15 and 16, it is interesting to note that virtually all the environments measured exceeded the maximum levels recommended. The noise level of an office with ventilating equipment exceeds the recommendations for quiet, efficient work. Business machines also greatly increase annoyance. Household appliances particularly exceeded the recommended levels, since each increase in 10 PN decibels is equal to a doubling of the annoyance. (Decibel [dB] is the unit used to express noise intensity.) The recommended maximum PNL for the home is 53 PNdB; yet a food mixer, vacuum cleaner, dishwasher, or stove hood exhaust, each measuring over 80 PNdB, is almost ten times as annoying.

Of course, household equipment is not used continuously but over the course of the day, thereby lessening the effect. However, taken all together, the various pieces of equipment are used a great deal of the time; and the woman working on the job with annoying noise, who also vacuums, cooks, and washes in the home, will be more tired and hence probably will perceive noise as even more annoying. This is another potential health cost of the dual role of the modern working woman.

Noise and Stress

Exposure to noise can also be a source of physiological stress. In the previous chapter, the stress response (e.g., a

TABLE 15. SOME CRITERIA FOR PERCEIVED NOISINESS ON THE JOB

Presented are noise levels and perceived noise levels for several office situations, as well as homes and hospitals. Note that the noisy office with difficult telephone and speech communication is a typical application for secretarial spaces. These values should be compared to typical measured noise values tabulated in Table 16.

OFFICE NOISE	NOISE LEVEL [dB(A)]	PERCEIVED NOISE LEVEL [PNdB]	TYPICAL APPLICATION
1. Very quiet office—suitable for large conferences; telephone use possible	35	48	Executive office (50-person conference)
2. Quiet office—smaller conferences; telephone use possible	43	56	Private or semi-private office (20-person conference)
3. Office satisfactory for 6–8-foot table; normal voice here 6–12 feet	48	61	Medium office and industrial business office
4. Office satisfactory for 1–5-foot table; occasional slight difficulty in telephone use; normal voice 3–6 feet	55	68	Large engineering and drafting rooms
5. Unsatisfactory for conferences of more than 3; slightly difficult telephone use; normal voice 1–2 feet	63	76	Secretarial areas (italics supplied by author): typing, accounting areas, business machines
6. Very noisy and unsatisfactory	65	78	Not recommended
HOME NOISE	40	53	
HOSPITAL NOISE	40	53	

SOURCE: Adapted from Carl D. Kryter, *The Effects of Noise on Man* (New York: Academic Press, 1970), Tables 40 and 41.

TABLE 16. TYPICAL NOISE LEVELS AT HOME AND AT WORK

When comparing observed and recommended levels (Tables 15 and 16), it is important to remember that decibels are logarithmic. Every increase of 10 decibels is a 10-fold increase in intensity.

	NOISE LEVEL [dB(A)]	PERCEIVED NOISE LEVEL [PNdB]
OFFICE		
Conference Room		
With air conditioner	58	70
With fan only	52	62
Executive Office		
5 machines on	64	73
No machines on	46	52
Ventilating equipment on	47	53
Ventilating equipment off	40	41
HOME		
Garbage disposal	81	93
Typical vacuum cleaner	74	87
Dishwasher	70	82
Stove hood exhaust	75	88
Typical central-heating system	58	71

rise in blood pressure, increased heart rate, etc.) was related to social sources of stress. Noise is a physical source that can arouse the stress response as well, although it is still not clear what sound levels are needed for this arousal. Some people will respond to noise at levels that are not annoying to others, who need greater sound stimulation.

Various experiments have been conducted to explore the stress effects of noise; and some have shown that workers exposed to moderate and intense noise on the job have an increased incidence of circulatory, digestive, neurological, and psychiatric problems. Unfortunately, as we have already seen, the stress response can be elicited from many kinds of stressors; consequently, the results of studies like these are difficult to interpret. It must suffice to say that noise is a stressor and that the stress response and its potential adverse health effects represent another occupational health hazard to office workers and others whose job exposes them to noise.

Effects on Hearing Ability

Unless sounds are extremely loud, like a bomb blast, it takes time for permanent hearing loss to occur. At first, noise causes the delicate mechanisms of the ear to become traumatized, and a temporary shift in hearing ability develops. We have all experienced such temporary threshold shifts, as they are called. For example, after listening to a very loud rock band or riding in a very noisy car, you probably have felt an *immediate* loss of hearing ability, noticeable after leaving the noise source. Somehow you just could not perceive sound as well as before the noise exposure began. After a while, however, if you did not return to the noise but allowed your ears to rest, your normal hearing ability returned. The louder the noise and the longer the exposure, however, the longer the resting time necessary.

On the other hand, if noise exposure is frequent and there is insufficient time to allow the ears to rest in order to recover, the temporary shift will start to become a permanent hearing loss. Workers who function in very noisy environments usually do not have adequate recovery time, and their noise exposure is so great that permanent loss is almost inevitable. Some experts estimate that with workplace noise exposure, after about ten years on the job the permanent loss sustained will be about the same as the initial temporary loss.

Noise above 85 decibels can cause noise-induced hearing loss. Many women keypunch operators, laundry workers, hospital workers, and others work in surroundings and with equipment that exceed this level and that consequently are unsafe. Table 16 shows some of these jobs and gives examples of the noise associated with various pieces of equipment. It is interesting that there are many household appliances also listed which, in addition to the annoyance factors already listed, create an intense sound level that can be dangerous to hearing.

Of course, using a blender once in a while, for example, will not in itself cause hearing loss; but combined with all the other sources of noise pollution we face in our modern, industrial society, over the years some hearing loss is almost inevitable. Several studies have shown that people growing old in a noise-polluted society such as ours will suffer more hearing loss than those who grow old in a quiet, rural environment.

A women who is faced with noise on the job, when she commutes to work, and while she is doing her household chores will, of course, be exposed to a combination of noise insults, which can, and probably will, affect her hearing ability. Unfortunately, there is little data available that indicates the extent of hearing loss among women workers. Most studies have concentrated on men working in industrial surroundings. However, if a woman is exposed to noise, she too will suffer a loss of hearing.

It is interesting to note that women do seem to have superior hearing ability compared to that of men. Many people try to account for this by arguing that women are exposed to less noise than men are. However, in studies of men and women from similar work-exposure backgrounds, it has been shown that women's hearing ability compared to men's when matched for age, was still superior. No one understands why this is true or how this affects women's ability to withstand noise exposure. Long-term studies are needed.

In summary, noise is an annoyance; it impairs one's ability to work and communicate; it can elicit a physiological stress response in people who are exposed to it; and, of course, excessive noise exposure will permanently damage a person's ability to hear.

OFFICE AIR POLLUTION

The air in an office must be circulated and replenished with fresh air. It should flow quickly enough to keep the atmosphere clean, yet it should not cause drafts. Most buildings are inadequately designed for air, temperature, and climate control. They are either too hot or too cold or too humid or too dry—and, of course, in a new office building, one can almost never open a window. The various aspects of stress in the controlled environment of an office building are not duly appreciated when the buildings are first designed.

However, recirculated air in an office can also be a source of disease. Sometimes improperly maintained air conditioning systems will breed spores and funguses, which are circulated through the air and can lead to cold-like irritations and allergies. In some buildings, asbestos, which is used to insulate the ducts and the building itself, becomes exposed and floats in the air. Because the inhalation of asbestos fibers can cause cancer, as well as other lung disease, especially if the exposed worker smokes, there should be no unnecessary exposure to this mineral. Asbestos that is carried home on the clothes can also adversely affect family members. Although it is unlikely that office levels will be that high if there is any evidence of a white dust settling in the office, it should be immediately determined whether it is asbestos.*

Office copying machines, cleaners, and liquids are other sources of chemical air pollution. The power source in an electronic stencil machine produces ozone, an extremely irritating chemical (see pages 100–2), and the light source of dry copiers emits ultraviolet radiation. Excessive eye exposure to ultraviolet light can lead to the formation of

* The federal Occupational Safety and Health Administration (OSHA) can help with this. Local offices are listed in the telephone directory under U.S. Government, Department of Labor.

cataracts, but there is no available data as yet on the degree of exposure in an office situation and the risk involved. The studies just have not been done. Other chemical hazards are listed in Table 14.

Office work also presents many safety hazards, as several surveys that have found a rather alarming rate of occupational accidents and injuries will testify. One projection of the annual rate among the 25–30 million office workers is 40,000 disabling injuries and more than 200 deaths.[9]

Some of the details on the accident rate are shown in Table 17, which is based on a five-year study of about nine thousand employees in a large New York life insurance company. Falls from chairs, escalators, stairs, etc., were the

TABLE 17. TYPICAL OFFICE ACCIDENTS AND INJURIES IN ONE STUDY

CAUSE OF INJURY	NUMBER
Falls or slips on walking surfaces (941)	
Slippery surface	245
Large objects in path	164
Uneven surface	105
Small objects (litter) in path	55
Fainting, seizure	30
Loss of balance in pushing/pulling object	14
Unspecified	328
Falls or slips on stairs or steps (384)	
Uneven surface	133
Slippery surface	15
Littered surface	5
Unspecified	231
Falls or slips from chairs	192
Falls or slips from elevation (76)	
Standing on office furniture (including chairs)	31
While climbing ladders	24
Other	21
Falls when entering or leaving elevators	10

SOURCE: U. S. Department of Labor, *Job Safety and Health* (Washington, D. C., February 1976).

greatest source of accidents, followed by disabling injuries that come from lifting office equipment, or working with office machines. File cabinet drawers and kick stools constitute other potential instruments of injury in the office. For example, if two drawers in a top-heavy file cabinet are opened simultaneously, the entire cabinet can tip over. Files should be bolted for stability. Also, although staple guns do not kill, the staples in protruding files can cause puncture wounds, which in turn can cause infection.

Retail Sales

Women whose work is in the area of retail sales generally are required to stand for many hours a day and often must reach for items on shelves and carry merchandise around. They also must deal with customers, some of whom will be carrying and transmitting infectious diseases. In addition, their jobs afford no privacy and little variation from day to day.

STANDING

There has been inadequate research on the health effects of standing, especially with respect to varicose veins, which are dilated veins in the legs as shown in Figure 18. This is especially ironic, since about 40 percent of all women have varicose veins to some degree, and the majority of women workers either sit or stand for long periods, which, of course, affects circulation and varicosities.

When a person stands for some time, a great deal of pressure develops in the blood vessels of the legs, and the veins become dilated, especially if the muscular vein walls have already been weakened by circulatory stresses like pregnancy or excess weight. Some authorities think that the extra pressure of standing or weight bearing can also lead to a weakening of the muscular walls of the veins.

If the varicose veins are uncomplicated and the valves that control the blood flow in the veins have not been

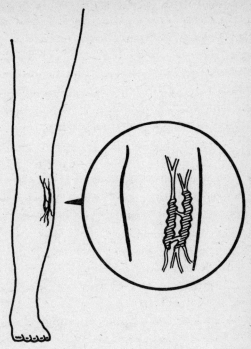

Figure 18. VARICOSE VEINS

damaged, the dilated veins will respond and improve with the use of support stockings. If the structure of the veins has been badly damaged, however, then painful complications like swelling, blistering, skin ulcers, and rash may develop. These conditions should receive medical attention, since severe cases must sometimes be treated surgically.

The reduced blood flow caused by the pooling and dilation of the blood in the legs to the feet from standing can also lead to swelling of the feet and ankles. The thigh muscles may become strained, fatigued, and painful as well.

All these problems can be alleviated by avoiding excessive standing, which is the usual medical advice given. It is not very useful advice, however, to a woman whose livelihood depends on a job that requires much standing. These jobs must be redesigned so that workers can sit down regularly and can rotate away from jobs in which sitting is not feasible. Unfortunately, in many jobs like sales clerking, if a worker is sitting, it gives the impression that she is doing nothing or that sales are slow; consequently, she is required to pay a health penalty for keeping up "good appearances." Thus, even though ebbs in the flow of customers are to be expected, there still may not be any facility for sitting down. Keeping up "good appearances" is surely a matter of social definition, which can be redefined for better health.

Another "good appearance" ruling that is detrimental to health is the wearing of panty girdles. Girdles impede the blood flow and can aggravate all the effects of standing. It is also standard medical advice to avoid wearing girdles if one has varicose veins. Some department stores and other places of employment either explicitly or implicitly require the use of binding corsetry of their employees because it gives them a "better" appearance. This is adding insult to the injury of jobs that require standing. Wearing girdles is a custom that for many women, in the author's opinion, should be more honored in the breach than the observance, especially if a woman's job entails standing.

It is essential to relieve the strain on muscles and circulation that comes from too much standing or sitting. A rest from standing is comfortable sitting, while a rest from sitting is standing or walking around. Jobs must be designed so that a person is not required to assume any one posture for long lengths of time. Muscles have a remarkable ability to recover if they are allowed to rest, and they recover better if there are several short periodic rests rather than one extended rest after a long period of stress.

Rest periods are another solution to the problem of mental fatigue that so often is a part of women's usual occupations. As we have already noted, mental fatigue will be translated into muscular fatigue as time goes on. This will worsen the muscular effects of prolonged sitting or standing.

Working with the public probably increases the risk of contracting communicable diseases. Although there really have not been any definitive studies on this, it seems reasonable that the more people a person comes in contact with, the more likely she is to contract an illness like the flu or a cold. Dealing with the public is also stressful and emotionally demanding, as has been noted previously.

Service and Domestic Work

Many of the hazards facing service workers like hotel chambermaids, hairdressers, and waitresses have already been discussed. Standing, bending, lifting, and carrying, for example, are universal problems. Contact with infected objects like laundry and dishes is a source of disease similar to those of hospital work. The stress aspects of the job—emotional fatigue, dealing with the public, or insufficient wages—are social sources of stress that have been dealt with in Chapter Two.

SKIN DISEASES

One health problem common among people in the service industries is skin disease. Because so much of the work involves frequently wetting the hands and/or coming into contact with chemicals, the skin is directly affected. Skin disease is the leading industrial disease in the United States today. This partially results from the fact that unlike many other occupational diseases which can remain hidden for years or which may be attributed to other causes, skin diseases are easily noticed. Working people can also often relate the onset of the symptoms to exposure to particular conditions at work.

The skin, as shown in Figure 19, consists of two layers covered by a tough material that is resistant to many dusts, germs, and chemicals. The inner layer contains hair follicles, blood vessels, sweat glands, and glands that produce a protective wax. The outer layer, the wax, and a layer of nonliving cells act as a barrier, guarding the inner skin layer and the rest of the body from harmful physical and chemical agents.

Many industrial chemicals and cleaning solvents can dissolve the wax in the skin, resulting in different degrees of

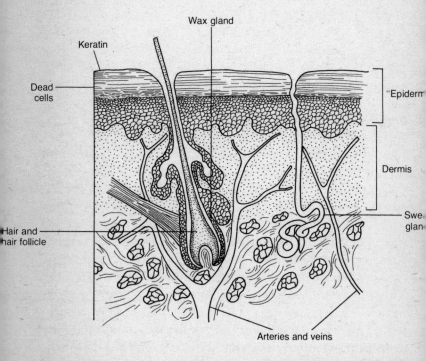

Figure 19. MICROSCOPIC CROSS-SECTION OF THE SKIN

SOURCE: Jeanne Stellman and Susan Daum, *Work Is Dangerous to Your Health* (New York: Pantheon, 1973).

skin irritations, or dermatitis. These range from a mild reddening of the skin or perhaps reddening with cracking to extreme cases in which the skin may develop oozing and crusting sores, which can become infected. Sometimes the hair follicles and wax glands become clogged, leading to acnelike conditions that may also become infected. Some chemicals cause the skin to darken; others cause it to lose color. And finally, a comparatively large number of industrial chemicals can lead to the formation of skin growths, which may be either cancerous or benign.

While some substances affect the skin by irritating it, others can produce allergic skin reactions, which are sometimes called hypersensitivity, or contact dermatitis. People who handle foods, such as fish, fruits and vegetables, vanilla and cinnamon; who use soap containing germicidal agents; who work in the plastics and rubber industries; or who handle ointments and cosmetics, as well as certain hair dyes, are likely to be exposed to skin-sensitizing agents. Contact dermatitis looks like the dermatitis caused by irritating substances; however, while everyone who comes into contact with irritating substances like acids will be affected by them, only some persons will develop contact dermatitis from those chemicals that cause skin allergies.

For example, not everyone is allergic to poison ivy—in fact, some people can handle it without any reaction. Another example is hay fever. Although some people are severely affected by certain pollens, others are not. About 20 percent of the work force can be expected to develop allergic contact dermatitis if they come into contact with sensitizing chemicals. Sometimes a person can work with a substance for many years and suddenly develop an allergy to it. This can be a major problem to a woman who has put many years of service into a job. If there is no way to avoid the allergy-producing agent, she may be forced to leave her job; and unless there is some other work available within the company, she may lose many years of seniority (if she has seniority from belonging to a trade union), a pension, advanced job status, and so on. Some chemicals that can cause skin diseases and that are encountered in jobs held by women, especially in personal services and cleaning positions, are listed in Table 18.

Physical conditions on the job can also affect the skin. Women who must wet their hands often, especially if they come into contact with harsh detergents or chemicals at the

TABLE 18. SOURCES OF SKIN DISEASE ON THE JOB

I. Leading jobs for skin disease: One ten-year survey of 1,752 patients with occupational dermatitis found that hospital work and cleaning accounted for 55 percent of all cases. The top twelve occupations for women are listed.

1. Hospital	7. Rubber industry
2. Hospital cleaning	8. Plastics industry
3. Cleaning	9. Textile industry
4. Hairdressing	10. Laboratory
5. Food industry	11. Nursery/florist
6. Hotel/restaurant	12. Housework

SOURCE: S. Fregert, "Occupational Dermatitis in a Ten-Year Survey," *Contact Dermatitis* 1 (1975); 96–107.

II. Examples of typical sources of skin irritants and allergies[a]

Irritation

Soaps	Phenolic compounds and other disinfectants
Cleaning compounds	Strong alkalis, bleaches, solvents

Allergies

Food handling	Fruits and vegetables
	Flavoring agents: vanilla, cinnamon
	Conditioners and bleaches in flour
Textile work	Formaldehyde
Hospital work	"Caine"-type skin anesthetics and skin antihistamines
Dishwashing	Fungus infection of nails
Offset printing	Cobalt and chromium in work
Rubber and plastics industry	Epoxy resins, catalysts, anti-oxidants, and accelerators

Increased skin susceptibility

Machine operation	Friction, pressure, trauma, or vibration
	Sunlight

[a] See, e.g., Jeanne Stellman and Susan Daum, *Work Is Dangerous to Your Health* (New York: Pantheon, 1973) for a more complete listing.

same time, can develop irritating skin reactions and even a fungus infection of the nails. A person whose hands, whether wet or dry, are exposed to heat or cold can also develop a skin reaction. Cold weather or cold water, depending on the amount of exposure, can cause mild injuries and lead to rashes, blisters, or, in extreme cases, open wounds. On the other hand, high temperatures can produce skin reactions like prickly heat, which can also become an open, oozing wound, especially in people who are overweight and have poor sweat-control mechanisms. The body and the skin cannot adjust to temperature extremes. Other effects of temperature extremes will be discussed later in this chapter.

If the skin is broken by cuts or scrapes, or from handling vibrating tools, its ability to act as a protective barrier is vastly diminished. Bacteria and other infectious agents can invade, leading to infection.

The last kind of skin disease to be discussed here is skin cancer. Most forms of skin cancer do not spread quickly, so that with early diagnosis, the growths can be removed with no apparent long-term danger. Soot and some oils and greases can cause skin cancer, especially in conjunction with exposure to sunlight or ultraviolet radiation. People who work with any of these chemicals or who work outdoors should have regular medical checkups specifically directed toward looking for signs of skin disease and cancer.

Preventing Skin Disease

The vast majority of skin diseases and injuries can be prevented by avoiding direct contact with chemicals, prolonged wetting of the hands, and injuries. Unfortunately, the requirements of many jobs too often run counter to this common-sense advice. If employees must work with chemicals, there are several protective steps that should be taken:

1. *Good hygiene*: Wash-up time and good facilities for cleaning should be allotted to people whose hands are exposed to chemicals. Abrasives, powders, solvents like turpen-

tine, harsh soap powders, all make cleaning up quicker but can be as harmful as, or more harmful than, the conditions that originally dirtied the hands. If enough time is provided for people to keep their hands clean with mild soap—several times a day if necessary—much disease could be avoided. Lanolin-containing lotions should also be available to replace the oils and fats in the skin that have been lost.

If it is really impractical to wash up during the day, there are "waterless" cleaners that can be used until it is convenient to do a complete soap-and-water washup.

2. *Substitution of chemicals and processes*: Wherever possible, the least irritating chemicals should be used. If mechanical equipment, such as vegetable slicers or mop squeezers, is available, it should be used so that hand contact is avoided.

3. *Good housekeeping*: Management should maintain good housekeeping techniques to eliminate all unnecessary exposure to dusts, fumes, and chemicals in the workplace. Sufficiently large work crews should be maintained to keep the workplace clean and in good operating condition.

4. *Protective equipment*: In some cases, it may be possible to wear protective gloves, as, for example, with a chemical or procedure that is used only from time to time. Many people find it very difficult to wear gloves for long periods, however, because the gloves are uncomfortable and cause their hands to perspire. Perspiration and poor air circulation in the gloves also can irritate skin and make it even more susceptible to damage if it comes into contact with chemicals. Chemicals that are caught inside gloves are more dangerous than is direct contact with them because gloves keep them in close contact with the skin. To eliminate this potential problem, gloves should reach at least one third of the way up the arm. Workers who are required to wear gloves should be given frequent periods during which they can remove the gloves, allowing perspiration to evaporate.

Laundry Work

The work was now under full blast, and every one of the hundred and twenty-five girls worked with frenzied energy as the avalanche of clothes kept falling in upon us and were sent with lightning speed through the different processes, from the tubs to the packers' counters. Nor was there any abatement of the snowy landslide—not a moment to stop and rest the aching arms.

—Dorothy Richardson, *The Long Day*[10]

New machines with larger capacities and higher operating speeds are constantly being introduced and these often present increased hazards . . . as follows: crushing of fingers . . . entanglement of hair . . . arm amputation . . . trapping of fingers or hands . . . scalding . . . falls . . . electric shock . . . fires . . . explosions. . . . In the absence of adequate ventilation, the environmental conditions can be very unhealthy and tiring, especially in hot and humid climate conditions.

—International Labor Organization,
*Encyclopedia of Occupational Health
and Safety*[11]

Laundering dirty linens and clothing can be a dangerous, unpleasant job. Laundry workers are exposed to infectious diseases in hospitals and to hazardous industrial chemicals in facilities that wash work clothes. Working in a laundry involves standing all day, sometimes on wet or damp floors, as well as exposure to a hot, humid environment. In addition, the equipment in most laundries is very noisy and presents safety hazards to operators. This combination of factors, along with relatively low wages and no social prestige, makes laundry work difficult, tiring, and unhealthy for the more than 250,000 women engaged in it.

THE HOT ENVIRONMENT

Working in a hot environment, especially a humid one like a laundry, is not only uncomfortable—it is unhealthy. Humans are comfortable only in a rather narrow temperature/humidity range, averaging 73° F. with a relative humidity of 45 percent. The more a person exerts herself, the more heat her own body generates and, therefore, the lower the external temperature needed for comfort. Unfortunately, many jobs like laundry work, which require heavy physical activity, are jobs whose environments have excessively high temperatures—the opposite condition from what is necessary for health and comfort.

The body's chemical reactions generate heat, which the body dissipates by several mechanisms. For example, most of the body's heat is lost by the evaporation of sweat. Energy (heat) is required in order for the water in sweat to evaporate from the skin surface. High temperatures, however, tax the body's ability to dissipate heat, for if the outside temperature is high, the environment will be contributing its energy to the evaporation of the sweat. Less heat will have left the body because less body heat was used. It is also necessary for the body to maintain an internal temperature of about 98.6° F. High temperatures can seriously interfere with this function and can lead to strain on the heart. In extreme cases, this can be fatal.

When workers are regularly exposed to hot environments, their bodies try to adapt, or *acclimatize,* to them. This involves changes in perspiration patterns and blood circulation. In order to lose heat most efficiently, the blood vessels in the skin dilate. When a person is accustomed to heat, the body learns to balance the blood distribution for maximum heat loss with minimum effect on the internal organs. In people unaccustomed to heat, the dilation of the blood vessels is compensated for by the constriction of vessels to the kidney, liver, and digestive organs. However, in extreme cases, the liver can be damaged by receiving insufficient oxygen and blood.

Sweat-gland operation is also changed during acclimatization. People unused to heat generally perspire in only a few places, like the armpits. But the body houses two and a half million sweat glands, many of which are normally not used. Acclimatization activates these glands. Of course, once a person perspires heavily and saturates her clothes, the sweat can no longer evaporate. Also, very humid air, as in a laundry, is already saturated with moisture, so that the sweat cannot evaporate. There is also the danger of perspiring so much that the body becomes dehydrated, which can lead to shock. Salt pills or salty foods can help prevent this, as can acclimatization. A young and healthy person may be able to acclimatize well, but older people or those with circulatory problems may never be able to adjust to hot environments.

Just because the body can acclimatize to heat does not mean that there are no long-range effects of heat exposure. It simply means that there are no immediate acute effects, such as heat shock or heat stroke. But the strain on the heart and on circulation remains. It is unclear what the health costs of heat stress are because the research has not been done. Since heart and circulatory disease are the most prevalent diseases in society, however, it is reasonable to assume that heat stress can contribute to such disease. Also, acclimatization is not permanent. It takes between four and six days on the job to acclimatize and about one week off the job to lose between one third and one half of the body's ability to adapt to heat. After an absence of about three weeks from heat exposure, the body has returned to normal and will have to begin all over again to adjust to heat.

Hot environments, as well as cold environments, are sources of stress. Just as noise exposure can cause the body to undergo the stress response, so, too, can heat act as an environmental stress. Although long-range studies have not been carried out, it seems reasonable to expect that stress, with its strain on the circulatory system and the heart, will intensify the other effects of heat exposure on the body.

CONTAMINATION

We have already discussed the dangers of infection from contaminated objects (see pages 93–94), but laundry workers will also be exposed to toxic dusts and chemicals if they launder work clothes. For example, cases of a rare, fatal cancer—mesothelioma—which is caused by asbestos dust, were found among women who laundered their husband's asbestos-contaminated work clothes. Laundry workers who are exposed to similar contaminants, probably in higher concentrations, will also be at risk for disease. Some English laundry workers who were exposed to the pottery dust of pottery workers' clothing, for example, were observed to develop lung diseases.

It is obvious that there should be an enclosed vacuuming procedure for dust-contaminated work clothes and a disinfecting process for potentially infected linens. Now that laundered work clothing must be supplied as a mandated part of some occupational health standards, like the asbestos-exposure standard promulgated by the Occupational Safety and Health Administration (OSHA), the exposure of large numbers of laundry workers to industrial toxins is inevitable. Laundries must take adequate and essential precautions immediately.

SAFETY HAZARDS

Much of the equipment that is used in the laundry industry—like washing machines, manglers, and extractors—can cause serious, permanent injury and even death if they are improperly designed and maintained. For example, it is common for laundry sterilizing equipment not to be equipped with safety locks which prevent the doors from being opened while there is still steam inside. Many of the manglers, which iron sheets and other flat laundry, and other rotary equipment are not fitted with guards to keep a worker's fingers and hands from being caught, crushed, or

TABLE 19. HAZARDS OF LAUNDRY WORK

Heat Stress	The hot and humid environment is a serious cause of stress and can adversely affect the heart and circulatory system, especially in unacclimatized workers. Rest periods and climate control are essential.
Noise	The high noise levels found can lead to permanent hearing loss. Rest periods and engineering control are essential.
Irritating Chemicals	Soaps, bleaches, and disinfectants all have severe effects on skin, especially if hands are wet.
Infection and Exposure to Toxic Chemicals	Contaminated clothing and linens can be a serious source of hazards. Pre-vacuuming and isolation practices should be instituted.
Mechanical Injury	Unguarded laundry equipment like manglers and extractors should be modified. Frayed electrical wires should be repaired. Safety locks and switches are also essential to prevent contact with steam or still operating equipment.
Physical Stress	Excessive standing, lifting, bending, and carrying can lead to back strain and other musculo-skeletal problems.
Accidents	Wet slippery floors are a hazard.

amputated. Often the equipment does not have automatic shutoff devices for emergencies, so that if a limb is accidentally caught in the machine, it will inevitably be injured.

The electrical grounding of laundry equipment is also often inadequate. This is particularly dangerous, since laundry work of course uses water, a highly conductive substance. The pressure vessels and steam receivers in laundries are also sometimes poorly maintained so that there is danger from explosion. These hazards, as well as other safety and health hazards of laundry work, are described in Table 19.

Industrial Work

About 15 percent of all women workers work in industrial, blue-collar jobs, mostly in the textile and clothing industries. There are a large number of women, however, who work as inspectors, packers, and assembly-line workers, as we have already noted. More than 110,000 women work in the production of electrical and electronic equipment, and over 60,000 women are employed in the rubber and plastics industries.

Much industrial work involves exposure to toxic chemicals, dusts, fumes, and other hazards. Some of these, such as noise, heat, radiation, and skin disease, have already been discussed. Because of the wide range of occupational health hazards in industries where women work, it is not possible to deal with them in detail here. There are about 15,000 chemicals in use in industry today, and the number of new processes and products grows daily. This section will briefly summarize the types of hazards commonly found in industrial jobs filled by large numbers of women. Appendix I lists hazards often encountered in women's occupations, while Appendix II is a quick guide to the effects of the hazards detailed in the first appendix. For additional information on industrial hazards, the reader is referred to other sources.[12] However, the effect of dusts and irritating or sensitizing chemicals on the lungs will be discussed here in some detail inasmuch as lung diseases constitute an important and substantial part of all occupational diseases.

OCCUPATIONAL LUNG DISEASES

The lungs are part of the respiratory system and perform the vital function of transferring oxygen from the air to the blood. Oxygen is, of course, essential to life, and no organ system can survive without it for long. The respiratory system consists of a major breathing tube, the trachea, or windpipe, which connects to the nose and the throat. This tube branches into two other main airways, the bronchi, one in each lung, which branch out further into medium-sized, then smaller, airways, the bronchioles. These tiniest airways end with delicate air sacs, alveoli, which resemble clusters of grapes. There are millions of such sacs throughout the lungs.

The air sacs are surrounded by tiny blood vessels. Oxygen from the air diffuses across the air-sac walls, which are one millionth of an inch thick, to be picked up by the red blood cells and transported around the body. If the air-sac walls become damaged, torn, or scarred, their ability to transfer oxygen is impaired, and ill health, such as heart disease or chronic bronchitis and emphysema, will result. Many substances encountered in the workplace can lead to such impairment. Figure 20 shows this process, and Table 20 details some of the substances.

IRRITATING SUBSTANCES

Substances like acids and alkalis give off fumes, which can irritate the respiratory system. The airways are lined with mucus-producing glands, like those in the nose. Mucus production is part of the body's natural defense mechanism. When the airways are irritated by foreign substances, the glands produce more mucus in order to dissolve the substances and remove them. If the irritation is frequent, such as from daily workplace exposure to industrial pollutants or heavy cigarette smoking, then the glands secrete a great deal of mucus and become swollen. This blocks the airways and, because the normal air flow of exhaling is impeded, can result in the development of a back pressure on the air sacs. This pressure can cause the delicate walls separating the sacs to break down or tear, a condition known as emphysema. The excess mucus also tends to become infected, leading to chronic bronchitis, which is characterized by a hacking, phlegm-producing cough. When chronic bronchitis and emphysema develop, the oxygen that does pass across the walls is limited, and the air and fluid in the lungs become stale and more prone to infection, another source of damage to air-sac walls. A vicious cycle of disease has set in.

Women who work in the electronics industry, in manufacturing, or in packing may be exposed to a variety of

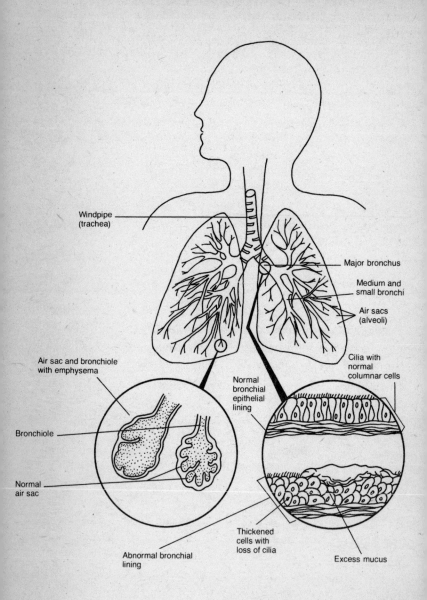

Figure 20. THE LUNGS AND LUNG DISEASE

TABLE 20. OCCUPATIONAL LUNG DISEASES

ACUTE REACTIONS: Generally characterized by fluid in the lungs (pulmonary edema); may be followed by pneumonia and permanent lung dysfunction. Acute reactions may be caused by overexposure to substances like

> halogens: chlorine, bromine, iodine
> nitrogen oxides
> ozone
> phosgene
> soldering fumes
> strong acids (e.g., hydrochloric)
> strong bases (e.g., ammonia)
> welding fumes

CHRONIC REACTIONS: Dust diseases (pneumonconioses): Inorganic dusts cause scarring and hardening of lung tissue (fibrosis). Some specific dusts are

> asbestos
> carbon black
> coal dust
> mineral wool, rock wool fibrous glass*
> silica
> talc

ALLERGIC RESPONSES: Organic dusts may contain plant fibers, fungi, or bacteria, and produce an allergic-like reaction. These ducts include

> cedar
> detergent enzymes
> cotton dust, flax, hemp (brown lung or byssinosis)
> molds and fungi in air conditioning systems
> moldy hay and other vegetable products (farmers' lung)
> mushroom spores (mushroom pickers' lung)
> redwood sawdust
> sugar cane fibers (bagassosis)

CHRONIC BRONCHITIS AND EMPHYSEMA: Can be the end result of many long-term low-level exposures to irritating dusts and gases, and to cigarette smoke.

---

* Animal effects observed.

substances that can irritate the lungs. Acids, alkalis, and some dusts are all irritants. The fluxes and other fumes that are part of the soldering process are also sources of irritating fumes.

Cosmetologists and hairdressers, who are exposed to

sprays and lacquers all day on the job, have been found to develop lung dysfunction. Aerosols are particularly hazardous because they contain extremely small droplets suspended in the air and can effectively make their way deep into the respiratory tract, where they can do the most harm.

DUSTS

Breathing fine dust particles in the air can also lead to lung disease. The airways are lined with very fine hairs called cilia, which serve to trap and sweep particles out of the airways. Very fine particles, however, do pass right through the cilia, possibly damaging them on the way. If the particles penetrate deep inside the airways to the air sacs, they can lodge there, causing the formation of hard scar tissue. They can rip the air-sac walls as well. Scarred, thickened walls, a condition called fibrosis, do not permit the adequate transfer of oxygen. In addition, both the expansion and contraction of the lungs are much more difficult when the sacs are thickened, so that breathing becomes a physical exertion. Asbestos and silica are examples of dusts that can scar delicate lung tissue.

ALLERGIC RESPONSES

I just started to smother after I had been working in the spinning room for a few years. My work began to slow down. The boss came around and told me I wasn't moving fast enough. I stopped taking a lunch break. But I still couldn't get my quota. It was all that cotton dust flying around. I couldn't breathe. I finally had to quit work five years early—no pension, no medical compensation, not even one of those sheets we were making.

—Flossie Strickland, a South Carolina textile worker[13]

Some dusts like cotton dusts, or chemicals like TDI (toluene-di-isocyanate), a component of polyurethane, can create a hypersensitivity, or allergic response, in the lungs, leading to an asthmatic-like reaction. Substances that are sensitizers cause the small airways to contract so that the air cannot readily leave the lungs. The air, forcing its way out of narrowed passages, produces the characteristic wheezing sounds of asthmatic breathing. If the allergic reaction occurs regularly, it can result in the same sort of back pressure just described, causing the air-sac walls to tear and become emphysematous.

Scientists have shown that even if a chronic bronchitis or emphysema syndrome, or an asthmatic response, does not develop, people who are exposed to substances like cotton dust may develop a permanently decreased lung capacity. The mechanisms behind this are not well understood. There are thousands of cases of cotton-dust-induced lung disease, called brown lung, or byssinosis, among textile workers exposed to large quantities of the dust. At least a quarter of a million women are exposed to this substance.

The problems of allergies in industry are not confined to cotton dust. We have already discussed allergic skin reactions and listed some of the agents that women may work with that cause contact dermatitis. Other pulmonary allergens are the spores found in mushrooms. Thousands of women earn their livelihood from picking mushrooms, and many of these workers seem to be developing symptoms similar to those of the brown-lung victims. Chicken pluckers and other animal handlers can become sensitized to substances in their workplaces as well.

Scientists are also confirming that many substances that are known to cause skin allergies can also induce allergic lung responses. Some women in the textile and clothing industries who work with permanent-press materials have become allergic to the formaldehyde used to make the finish, and they have subsequently developed dermatitis. Recently, researchers noted that allergic responses can be induced in the respiratory system as well.

People who routinely smoke cigarettes expose themselves to irritants and particulate matter and, in so doing, are at greater risk of developing lung and heart disease. When a worker smokes and is exposed to substances that also cause such disease, the risk of sickness, disability, and death multiplies.

This discussion and the tables show that hundreds of thousands of women, like their working male counterparts, are exposed to substances and conditions that are dangerous to their health.

CHAPTER FOUR
WORK, REPRODUCTION, AND HEALTH

The course of nature with respect to pregnancy is so well known as to require no expatiation. . . . There are many burdens involved in the bearing and raising of children, which must be borne by those who take on that responsibility. . . . In the matter of pregnancy there is no way to find equality between men and women. The Great Creator so ordained the difference, and there are few women who would wish to change the situation. . . .

—Utah Supreme Court, February 4, 1975[1]

THE PROPAGATION of the human race depends on a large number of women fulfilling their social function of bearing children. Women who are pregnant are in a different physiological state than nonpregnant women, so that they may react differently to workplace conditions. Experiences such as the thalidomide birth-defect disaster illustrate that drugs, diet, and the pregnant woman's environment can seriously affect the developing fetus. Thus, working conditions at home and on the job are relevant to the health of the mother and child. This chapter will explore the health effects of work on pregnancy and childbirth.

It is paradoxical that although, as we have seen, woman's role has been so clearly defined in terms of her childbearing capacity, there exist no accurate statistics on how many women are employed during pregnancy or where they work. This is particularly distressful, since so many of the controversies about women in the workplace have dealt with potential risks for pregnant workers and their offspring. The lack of data again stems from the lack of recognition of women as workers and from the fact that few persons or institutions are seeking out the statistics. There has been only one major federal survey by the United States Public Health Service on work-force participation during pregnancy.[2] At the same time that the government is collecting massive amounts of health data from hundreds of thousands of people on a multitude of subjects, ranging from cancer to hearing loss to cuts and lacerations, its only survey on female employment during pregnancy was limited to about 4,000 women. It was carried out, in part, as a follow-up to an earlier British investigation that found that a woman's chance of producing a successful live birth was significantly lowered if she was employed during her pregnancy.[3]

Well-designed studies were much needed, as most earlier research was difficult to interpret. Medical and socioeconomic factors, such as diet, prenatal care, general health, and hygiene, had not been adequately accounted for. For example, in the British study just cited, it was author Alice Stewart's opinion that among the women she studied, the group that did not "work" were housewives engaged in housework no less demanding than the work of the employed women; yet these women were apparently more able to produce live children than women employed outside their homes. Perhaps this was the result of the employed women's carrying out two jobs—home and paid work. That possibility was not explored.

While Stewart reported an increase in the percentage of pregnancies that did not come to term among the employed women, she could find no other trends of complications due to employment. There was no significant increase in the number of birth defects, underweight infants, or complications of pregnancy and delivery. In sum, the results were puzzling.

Thus, while the intention of the survey was to clarify

previous findings, especially the effects of work on unsuccessful pregnancies, the survey itself was limited to women who had borne *live* children, and, in fact, unsuccessful pregnancies were excluded from the design entirely. The results therefore could neither confirm nor refute conclusions on the effects of employment on the ability to bear live children. In addition, the survey did not assemble any data on the type of work a woman did if she was employed during her pregnancy. Although the mother's employment history was not taken, incredibly the occupation of the *husband* was surveyed. The relevant part of the questionnaire is reproduced in Figure 21.

Despite the obvious drawbacks, the Public Health survey did reveal that a significant percentage of women worked at some time during their pregnancy. Here are some of the figures:

1. Fifty-nine percent of all women bearing a first child were employed.

2. Twenty-two percent of all women bearing a second or later child were employed.

3. About 50 percent of these women were employed at least until their seventh month of pregnancy.

4. As the woman's educational attainment level increased, so did the employment rate. Eighty-two percent of all pregnant college graduates were employed during their pregnancy. For second or later births this rate dropped to the same as all women—20–24 percent.

5. As family income increased, so did the woman's employment rate; but again, this was only for pregnancies leading to first-born children.

Table 21 gives some of the specific figures derived from the study.

Inasmuch as 1971 employment rates for women have continued to increase, particularly among women with children under the age of six, the number of women work-

PART II. RELATED INFORMATION

1. Were you employed outside your home at any time during your recent pregnancy?

☐ YES *(Answer a and b below)*   ☐ NO *(Go on to Question 2)*

    a. Did you work full-time at all during your recent pregnancy?

    ☐ YES   ☐ NO

    When did you stop working full-time?

Month	Day	Year
		19____

    b. Did you work part-time at all during your recent pregnancy?

    ☐ YES   ☐ NO

    When did you stop working part-time?

Month	Day	Year
		19____

2. What was the highest grade (or year) of regular school that you ever attended?
(Circle highest grade attended)

NONE------------------ 0

ELEMENTARY SCHOOL---- 1 2 3 4 5 6 7 8

HIGH SCHOOL---------- 1 2 3 4

COLLEGE-------------- 1 2 3 4 5 6+

Did you COMPLETE this grade?   ☐ YES   ☐ NO

3. What was the highest grade (or year) of regular school that your husband ever attended?
(Circle highest grade attended)

NONE------------------ 0

ELEMENTARY SCHOOL---- 1 2 3 4 5 6 7 8

HIGH SCHOOL---------- 1 2 3 4

COLLEGE-------------- 1 2 3 4 5 6+

Did he COMPLETE this grade?   ☐ YES   ☐ NO

4. Was your husband employed at the time of your child's birth?

☐ YES ⟶ Was he working *(check one)*   ☐ FULL-TIME?

☐ NO   ☐ PART-TIME?

5. What kind of work was your husband doing at the time of your child's birth? *(If he was not working then, please give information for his last job)*
GIVE FULL DESCRIPTION *(For example: grocery clerk, auto mechanic, elementary school teacher)*

_____

_____

_____

6. What was the total income of your family during 1962? *(Include all income such as wages, salaries, unemployment compensation, help from relatives, etc., received by all members of the family living with you when your baby was born)*

☐ NONE   ☐ $4,000 - $4,999

☐ UNDER $1,000   ☐ $5,000 - $6,999

☐ $1,000 - $1,999   ☐ $7,000 - $9,999

☐ $2,000 - $2,999   ☐ $10,000 - $14,999

☐ $3,000 - $3,999   ☐ $15,000 OR OVER

7. Where did you live when your baby was born?
(Please give your home address)

Number and Street
City (town) and State
County

Is this place on a city lot (or in an apartment building)?

☐ YES   ☐ NO

PHS-4425-19 *(page 3)*
4-63

_____

(Name and address of person completing this form)

Figure 21. A GOVERNMENT SURVEY ON PREGNANCY AND EMPLOYMENT

This reproduction of a page from a federal survey shows that while women were queried as to whether or not they worked during their pregnancies, only the occupation of their husbands was recorded.

SOURCE: U. S. Department of Health, Education and Welfare, *Employment During Pregnancy: Legitimate Live Births, U. S. 1963* (Washington, D. C.: U. S. Government Printing Office, 1963), p. 30.

TABLE 21. CHARACTERISTICS OF EMPLOYMENT DURING PREGNANCY

A 1963 Public Health Service survey of legitimate live births determined the distribution of employment patterns for a number of socioeconomic indicators.

	PERCENT DISTRIBUTION		
PERCENTAGE OF EMPLOYED MOTHERS	All Births	First Birth	Second and Higher Birth
By education			
Four years high school	32	70	21
1–3 years college	39	69	23
Four years college	30	70	14
By age			
Under 20 years	37	42	26
20–24 years	37	66	22
25–29 years	30	71	24
30–34 years	23	68	19
35+ years	22	—	21
By income			
Under $3,000	27	38	22
$3,000–4,999	30	53	21
$5,000–6,999	32	67	22
$7,000–9,999	37	81	24
Over $10,000	38	75	23
By employment pattern			
Full-time	23	47	18*
Part-time	6.1	5.5	6.5*
Full- and part-time	2.4	5.0	1.6*

* These data are for second-birth only.
SOURCE: U. S. Public Health Service, *Employment During Pregnancy* (Washington, D. C., 1968).

ing during pregnancy must also have increased greatly. Unfortunately, there is no accurate count of this taken by the various government bureaus so busily counting other population variables. In her excellent monograph "Occupational Health Problems of Pregnant Workers," Vilma Hunt calculates that in 1970 a conservative estimate is at least 1,000,000 infants out of the 3,718,000 legitimate children born were "exposed to a variety of work conditions

—safe and unsafe" before birth.[4] Given these great numbers of mothers and children, it is obvious that the lack of attention and interest in the health and welfare of pregnant workers and their offspring is truly an egregious example of the profound neglect that women as workers have suffered.

Biology of Reproduction

After the female reaches puberty, her body normally follows a complicated monthly cyclical process in which an egg (ovum, plural ova) is readied and released from her ovaries. If this egg is fertilized by a male sperm and successfully implanted in her uterus, under normal circumstances it will go through a long process of division, differentiation, and growth, eventually becoming a newborn infant.

The egg is derived from sex cells present in a female baby at birth. When a female is born, her ovaries already contain the starting cells of all her future eggs. The monthly ovarian cycle is devoted to secreting the hormones and the cells that cause the maturation and release of an egg each month as a potential candidate for fertilization. This process is called ovulation.

After ovulation has occurred, hormones continue to stimulate change and to prepare the uterus for receiving and nurturing the fertilized egg. In humans, as in all mammals, the developing animal grows in the mother's body in the uterus, in contrast to birds and reptiles, where development is external, in an egg. Part of the preparation of the uterus for pregnancy involves the thickening of uterine walls, dilation of glands, accumulation of water, and changing of the blood network. The uterus produces a substance called uterine milk, which is largely composed of nutrients. The milk is accumulated in the uterus as well and serves as an early food supply for the fertilized egg, or conceptus, just as the yolk in a chicken egg serves as the food supply for the hatchling (see Figure 22).

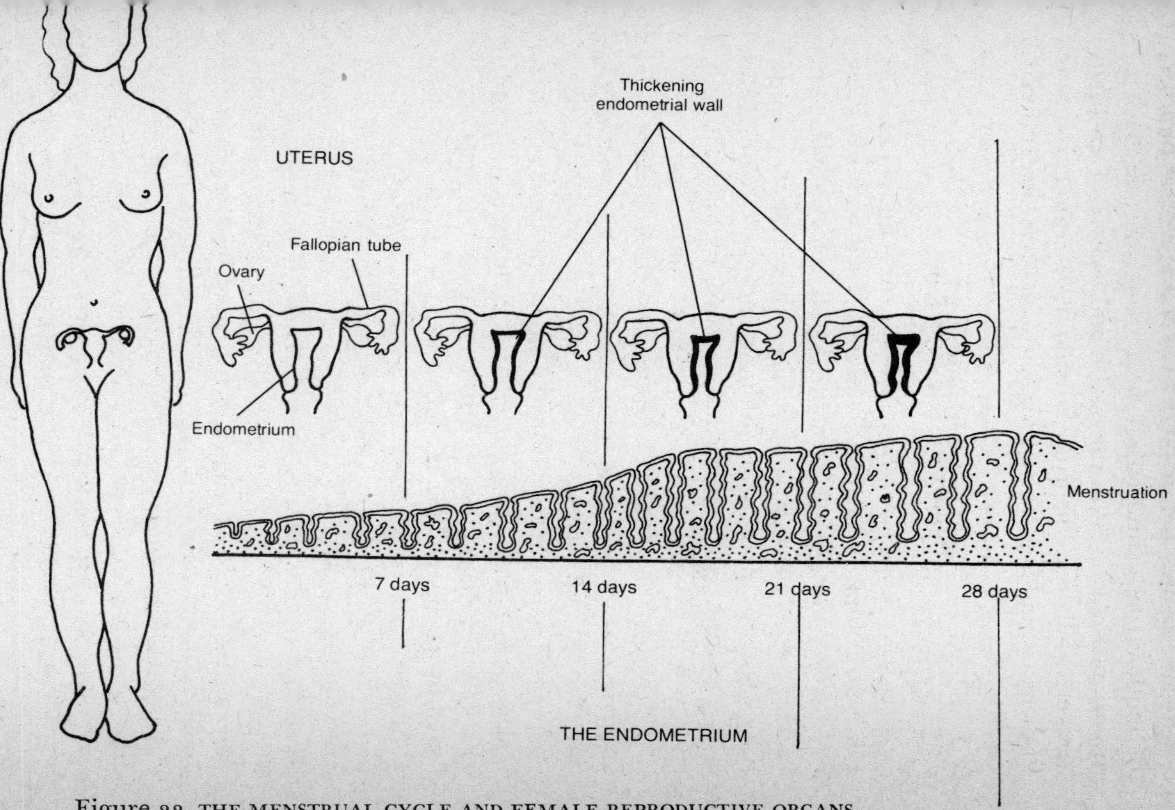

Figure 22. THE MENSTRUAL CYCLE AND FEMALE REPRODUCTIVE ORGANS

UTERUS

Fallopian tube

Ovary

Endometrium

Thickening endometrial wall

Menstruation

7 days

14 days

21 days

28 days

THE ENDOMETRIUM

[145]

If the egg is not fertilized, female hormone levels begin to drop, and the glands and other structures that developed in preparation for pregnancy collapse and shrink. Surface tissues die and vessels rupture, leading to hemorrhaging and discharge, the monthly menstrual cycle. Menstruation takes place about eleven to fourteen days after ovulation. After menstruation, the torn cells and glands regenerate themselves, and the process starts anew. If fertilization has occurred, the biological mechanisms that lead to the birth of a new human being, which the ovarian cycle has been preparing for, continue.

The first two steps of human reproduction thus are production of the sex cell and fertilization of the egg. Immediately after fertilization, the next step is the cleavage and reproduction of the fertilized egg into a small hollow sphere. Cells of different areas of this sphere have different future purposes and functions. One section will eventually give rise to skin cells, another to nervous system cells, and so on. The structure is still undifferentiated, however, and cannot in any way, shape, or form be even accidentally recognized as a human being. It is not even an embryo.

The process of growth and differentiation from a fertilized egg into an independent organism is an intricate one. Since all initial cells are identical, they have the potential of becoming any organ in any part of the body. Through a complex interaction of cellular, genetic, and environmental factors, the cells gradually differentiate themselves from one another in size, shape, and function. Soon they lose their ability to be interchanged, and their ultimate functional fate is determined.

The first eight weeks of growth and development are critical. It is during these eight weeks that all the organ systems are established. The period from the fourth week to the eighth week, inclusive, is called embryonic; from the third month to term it is called fetal. (The developing organism is an embryo and then a fetus, respectively.) The pre-embryonic and embryonic periods are the important times of organ differentiation. For example, at eight weeks the heart tissues and tubes are present; fingers and toes are formed; and the sex organ system cells are present.

It is essential to realize, however, that although organ *formation* of a three-month-old fetus is essentially complete, the fetus is still incapable of surviving outside the uterus because organ *function* has still not developed fully. For example, although the lungs are formed and there are small airways, air sacs have not yet grown, so the fetal lung cannot capture oxygen from the air, which would be necessary outside the womb. Although the guts are present, they are hollow, with no smooth muscles to make them operative. This is true of just about all the organ systems.

In other words, during the first eight weeks, a one-celled organism has grown and differentiated itself into a multi-celled fetus, and those cells are already devoted to different functions. The embryo is about one inch long and characteristically resembles a grown human. The critical period of development is nearly over, but there is no chance of survival in the world outside the mother.

It is generally not until the fetal age of twenty-eight weeks that a fetus can survive outside the uterus, though even then extraordinary medical intervention is necessary to keep it alive. A twenty-eight-week-old fetus, unlike the nine-month fetus, has inadequate temperature control; immature lung development; and insufficient calcium, iron, fat, and other reserves. A normal full-term infant makes up these deficiencies before birth. Though fetuses and newborns *resemble* adults, they are in no way miniature adults. Even after a normal birth, it is obvious that a newborn has few of the muscular and sensory capabilities of an adult. The relative proportion of head to body to limbs is different; hormonal secretions differ; and kidney, liver, and

digestive systems are incomplete. There is a long developmental distance between the fetal age of twenty-eight weeks
and the newborn infant and the mature adult.

The susceptibility of the egg, sperm, and fetus to damage
by toxic substances and conditions is, of course, of special
interest here. A fundamental principle is that susceptibility
varies with each stage of development just described (see
Figure 23).

The human organism is particularly susceptible to outside influences during the stages of organ development,
from about the eighteenth day to the sixtieth day after
conception, with the greatest sensitivity occurring between
the twentieth and thirtieth days. It should immediately be
obvious that many women do not *know* they are pregnant
at such an early stage, especially if they have generally
irregular menstrual periods. Of course, a woman who is
purposefully trying to become pregnant may soon be aware
of changes in her body that tell her she is pregnant well

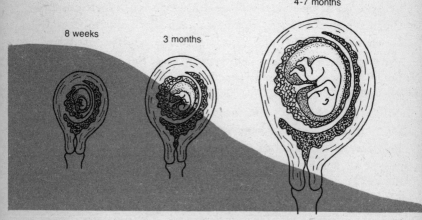

Figure 23. THE DECREASING SENSITIVITY OF THE
EMBRYO AND FETUS
The shaded background is a schematic representation of relative
sensitivity.

before her physician makes the news "official." A woman's awareness of pregnancy can be very early, particularly if she has already been pregnant or borne a child.

Given the intricacies of human development and the sensitivity of the embryo to outside influence, it is important to understand the environmental aspects of birth defects and the mechanisms by which the outside environment can affect the embryo and fetus within the mother.

Mutations

Teratology, a research area of continually growing interest, is the field of science that deals with birth defects. A mutation is a particular kind of birth defect, arising from alteration of the genetic material—genes and chromosomes —of the developing organism or from such alterations in the egg or sperm itself. The changes are permanent; and if the fetus survives and is born, its genetic makeup is permanently different. Genetic material is contained in biological structures called chromosomes. Humans normally have twenty-three pairs of matched chromosomes in the nucleus of every cell except sperm and egg cells. The nucleus of the sex cells carries only one of each of the twenty-three chromosomes. When fertilization occurs, the twenty-three chromosomes from the male sperm pair with the twenty-three chromosomes from the female to form a new set of twenty-three pairs of chromosomes (see Figure 24). A baby is thus the result of the combination of chromosomes from its mother and father, and its inherited characteristics will be a complex mixing of traits from each parent.

Not all changes in the genetic material occur in the sex cells before fertilization. Environmental factors, within the uterus and in the world afterward, interact with genetic heritage to produce the human whole. These factors, such as X-rays, can cause alterations in genetic material at any age, which, in turn, may be fatal to normal development. The embryo sometimes will fail to develop or will die

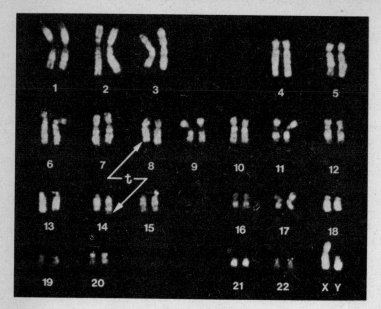

Figure 24. HUMAN CHROMOSOMES

The genetic material of human beings contains 23 pairs of matched chromosomes, which control growth and development. Scientists who study genetic effects isolate and grow certain human cells, which are examined microscopically, photographed, and enlarged. The chromosomes in the photograph have been cut out, paired, and arranged according to scientific custom. Abnormalities like breakage and re-arrangement can thus be observed. The "t" shows one translocation between the long arms of chromosomes 8 and 14. This translocation has been observed in patients with a rare cancer, Burkitt's lymphoma.

SOURCE: Barbara Kaiser-McCaw et al., "Chromosome 14 Translocation in African and North American Burkitt's Lymphoma," *International Journal of Cancer* 19 (1977): 482–86.

shortly after it is formed if the lethal mutation occurs soon after fertilization. If the sperm or egg is defective to begin with, fertilization may not take place, or the fertilized egg may not reach the embryo stage and simply be re-absorbed by the body. A more developed defective embryo may be aborted by the body; a defective fetus may be stillborn.

Other mutations can result in defects like Down's syndrome (mongolism), a relatively common birth defect, especially among the offspring of older parents. This mutation may be the result of the aging of the genetic material in the primary cells from which sex cells are derived. Since the primary cells are originally formed during organ development in the embryo, they age with the person and will be more fully ripened in an older individual. Until very recently, Down's syndrome was attributed to the aging of the female sex cells alone. Within the past several years, however, new analytical techniques have allowed closer examination of male sex cells, which are now known also to contain the dangerous extra chromosome responsible for the disease. The risk of mongolism consequently can no longer be attributed solely to older females as it was in the past.

The end results of most mutations that are not fatal before birth may not be obvious, since some of them may cause no discernible change or may produce subtle disorders, such as an error in a particular biochemical cell process. If a subtle abnormality rather than a gross structural defect like a deformed limb occurs, it can pass unnoticed for some time, possibly an entire lifetime. A mutation that occurs during the stage of organ differentiation or early organ development may result in an organ malformation. After about the eighth week, during the period of rapid growth, a mutation will generally retard growth or even arrest development entirely. A cleft palate, for example, occurs when upper palate growth has been arrested. During the last stages of fetal growth, or shortly after birth, mutations can be detrimental to the proper development of the functioning of organs and systems that are still immature.

Most birth defects cannot be neatly classified as due to one specific cause or another. Current estimates are that only about 20 percent of all defects are clearly carried on the genes, as is hemophilia, and about 5 percent are due to abnormalities carried in the genetic components. Most defects are attributed to complex environmental-genetic interactions, interactions that are poorly understood.

From a different perspective, we should realize that some mutations may be advantageous. The evolution of all species, human included, is the result of advantageous mutations over many millions of years. Advantageous mutations have become part of our total genetic heritage and have changed us from cave people into modern people. Unfortunately, the types of mutations we will be considering—generally arising from drugs, radiation, and chemicals —are probably not advantageous to human health and well-being. The end results of such mutations on the genetic inheritance of many generations hence are far from clear.

Problems in Discovering Mutations

One reason most end results are not obvious is that most outcomes of mutations do not affect gross development and may not be immediately perceptible at birth. The cause—a mutation—and the effect—the abnormality—will remain unidentified. As a purely hypothetical example, let us assume that a female hairdresser who inhaled six cans of vinyl-chloride-propelled aerosol hairspray vapors each working day produced defective offspring. (Remember, this is hypothetical.) However, the defects were not easily recognizable traits such as harelip. Instead, the mutation resulted in a subtle biochemical functional disorder leading to a high risk of developing leukemia. If one of her offspring did develop leukemia, that case of leukemia would be just one among thousands, since leukemia is not an exceptionally rare disease and its relationship to other environmental factors is not understood. Even if the inhalation of the spray did cause a mutation, and even if this mutation did lead to leukemia, it is easy to see how such an effect could remain undiscovered, hidden by a general prevalence of the disease in people with no history of parental exposure to large doses of aerosol vapors.

If there were thousands of people exposed to the spray and hence thousands of excess cases of leukemia in their offspring, *and* if astute medical practitioners took the appropriate history of parental occupational exposures, *and* if all the data were pooled and analyzed, then *perhaps* we could make an association of cause and effect.

Thalidomide: A Tragic Example

A good contrast is the tragic example of birth defects caused by thalidomide, a drug that produces a developmental defect in the embryo by somehow altering the paths of organ development (but not permanently altering the genetic material, like the previous example). This is another type of teratogenesis. For example, perhaps a drug or chemical interferes with a particular chemical reaction essential to the development of the nervous system. Although the embryonic chromosomal structures may be normal, sending normal control "messages" for nervous system development, the teratogen may be interfering with those message pathways, making normal development impossible.

The mothers of the 6,000–8,000 thalidomide babies born had been prescribed and had taken an apparently harmless drug, which, it was found, causes terrible birth defects, such as "seal limbs," where the deformed infant's hands are attached to the shoulders, and deformed ears. The relationship between thalidomide and the defects, however, could not be missed. First, the combination of these grotesque abnormalities is unique. Second, there were thousands of cases, immediately obvious at birth, so that attending physicians took extensive maternal medical histories, especially of drug exposures. All mothers had one thing in common: thalidomide usage. Sometimes they had taken the drug for only one day. Since the defects were so rare and since their appearance was not delayed until childhood or adulthood, they were clearly related to the development process. Despite this, thalidomide usage in Europe continued for many years, because the medical detective work involved was still very slow.

The horror of the tragedy of thalidomide babies illustrates several truisms about the nature and study of birth defects. To begin with, unless the defects are striking and obvious, they can easily go undetected. Also, thalidomide illustrates the great sensitivity of the embryo to environmental factors. Although it is a drug with little or no known toxicity either in human adults, or most species of test animals, it will almost always yield seriously defective human offspring if ingested by the mother between the twentieth and thirty-fifth day after conception. The only other animal species that show similar effects are some species of baboon and macaque monkeys. This was learned after the effects on humans were discovered. Routine animal testing, widely relied upon as an indicator of safe drug usage, could not predict the effects, because routine test animals were obviously not affected.

In sum, the fetus can be subject to congenital abnormalities from inborn defects arising from mutations or genetic transmissions, or from environmental factors that alter development and functioning. Unlike the thalidomide example, most defects result from a complex interaction of environment and heredity. The combination of extreme sensitivity of the embryo early in pregnancy and the growing worldwide environmental pollution both on and off the job may be taking its toll in birth defects, which, because of the scientific problems we have discussed, may not be discernible for many decades to come. Time will tell, and a great deal of prudence certainly couldn't hurt.

Between Mother and Child: The Placenta

During the first weeks of initial cell division, before the embryo stage, additional membranes that are not part of the embryo itself also begin to grow. These "extra-embry-onic" membranes will develop into the placenta, the organ that functions, in part, as a sort of membrane filter between the embryo and the outside world, represented largely by its mother's environment.

The function of the placenta is of importance to this discussion because all necessary nutrients, gases, and so on must pass across the placenta from the mother's blood to enter the fetal bloodstream. The placenta has other func-tions, like releasing hormones, but we will only be discussing its function as a membrane barrier between mother and fetus.

Unlike the bird egg, which is supplied with enough nutrients to sustain the chick embryo until it is hatched, the human egg has a scanty food supply available in its own structure and the uterine milk. Thus, very early in preg-nancy, development of the placenta proceeds so that the embryo can begin to receive its nourishment and support from its mother. From the outset the placenta is a mazelike network of fingerlike membrane projections. By about four weeks an umbilical cord structure from the embryo to the placenta has been formed. The umbilical cord has blood vessels that carry the diffused blood from the mother to the embryo, and venous structures, which return blood and waste products. It is a sort of supply lifeline, as shown in Figure 25.

The word "barrier" is not really a good one to describe the functions of the placental membranes, since almost all substances in the maternal bloodstream can pass through them. Some large entities like many bacteria are excluded, but other infectious agents like viruses can pass across the membrane. Most people are aware that German measles (rubella) causes serious birth defects if there is intrauterine exposure, especially within the first three months of devel-opment. Rubella is caused by a virus, which indeed passes across the placental membrane.

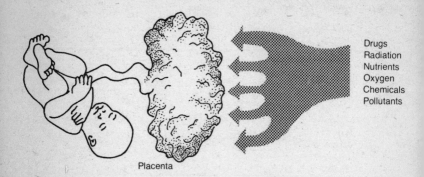

Figure 25. RELATIONSHIP BETWEEN FETAL AND
MATERNAL ENVIRONMENTS

Except for very large molecules or molecules bearing an electric charge, it is now thought that almost all foreign chemicals in the mother's blood, such as nicotine from cigarette smoke, can cross the placenta. There are differences in the rate of crossing, but essentially all pollutants that a pregnant woman has in her bloodstream will end up in the fetus. The process by which this crossing occurs is not actually understood very well; but even without an understanding of the mechanisms, it seems logical and prudent to assume that transfer will occur and to seek to prevent toxic substances with possibly harmful effects from entering the maternal bloodstream and therefore the fetus.

Reproductive Hazards: Offspring

Of the more than 15,000 chemicals in industrial and home use today, only relatively few have been tested for toxic effects on growth and development. There have also been very few large-scale studies of the effects on people and their offspring of exposure to most environmental pollut-

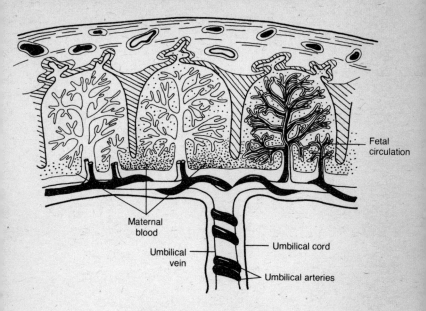

Figure 26. THE PLACENTA
Placental functions include the physiological exchange of oxygen, nutrients, water, and waste products, as well as the storage of nutrients and the production of hormones. Most substances in maternal blood can pass across the placenta, so that it does not act as a barrier.

ants. Physical workplace hazards, such as noise, vibration, radiation, and heat stress, are similarly unstudied and poorly understood. Table 22 is a compilation of data on reproductive hazards that are of occupational significance to women and that may be hazardous to normal childbearing. Some items in the table have been shown to adversely affect animals but not humans. The lack of human data, however, does not indicate safety but a lack of adequate research designed to answer the question of safety. Substances and conditions that have been found hazardous to humans so far are so marked in the table.

While it is obviously preferable to carry out tests and

TABLE 22. REPRODUCTIVE HAZARDS OF WORK: OFFSPRING

A list of common categories of hazards, with specific examples and occupations, where they can be expected to be found. Known teratogens like thalidomide are not included where they are not of occupational significance.

TYPE OF HAZARD	POTENTIAL HAZARDS	SOME OCCUPATIONS WHERE THEY OCCUR
Chemical hazards	Alkylating chemicals	Drug workers
	Anesthetic gases*	Operating-room personnel
	Dioxins	Chemical and pesticide workers
	Metals:	Battery-plant workers
	lead (?)	Electrical workers
	cadmium (?)	Dental workers
	copper (?)	Soldiers
	mercury (?)	
	Organic mercury compounds*	
	Pesticides: all types	
	Pesticides:	
	chlorinated hydrocarbon	Agricultural workers
	organophosphates	Microscopists (immersion oil)
	carbonates	Electrical workers
	arsenates	
	PCB's (polychlorinated biphenyls)*	
Irradiation and radioactive material	X-rays*	Dental technicians and assistants
	Radioisotopes*	Dentists
		X-ray technicians and radiologists
		Nuclear medicine technicians
		Some laboratory workers

Infections	Measles, chicken pox, German measles (rubella)*, hepatitis	Hospital workers—all phases Laboratory workers Teachers in contact with small children
	Herpes virus Toxic plasmosis Brucellosi Venereal disease	Animal handlers, meat cutters and inspectors
Insufficient oxygen supply (hypoxia)	Carbon monoxide and high-altitude chemicals, which affect blood (?) (See Appendix II)	Outdoor work: toll-booth operators, traffic-control workers, airline personnel
Physical hazards	Noise (?), heat (?), vibration, trauma	All types of industrial and service work
Cancer-causing substances (carcinogens) related to mutation (?)	Some aniline dyes	Drug workers, dye workers, some chemical lab workers; rubber workers
	MOCA, BCME, DES	Permanent-press workers and textile finishers Histology technicians
	Vinyl chloride	PVC plastics processors (?)

* Human effects observed.

discover potential ill effects of hazards from studying animals rather than by discovering adverse effects in humans, the problem is that people aren't rats, mice, guinea pigs, or rabbits. They are human beings, and their response to toxic substances will be uniquely human. Thus, the best that one can hope for is to avert disaster by observing effects in animals first and hoping that one has designed the experiment with enough insight and luck so that potential effects on humans will be observed.

It is evident that a number of workplace hazards which are potentially harmful to the developing embryo or fetus may be encountered by a sizable number of women at work. Hospital and health-care workers may be exposed to ionizing radiation and radioactive material, known to cause birth defects. Some infectious agents, like the rubella virus, which health-care workers as well as teachers and others who work with children are exposed to, are especially dangerous. Women exposed to rubella should be tested to determine if they are resistant and should be immunized if they are not. It is still not certain whether other infectious diseases, like hepatitis, can be harmful to normal human reproduction. Laboratory workers, meat processors, and other women who handle animals may be subject to many different and potentially harmful microorganisms.

Normal development may also be affected by the amount of oxygen and carbon monoxide in a woman's blood. Airline personnel, toll-booth operators, and other outdoor workers may have abnormal levels, especially if they also smoke.

Finally, exposure to various chemicals may present hazards to reproduction. Pesticides and mercury compounds are two such examples. A large number of women are also exposed to anesthetic gases. Women holding such positions as operating-room technicians and dental assistants are more likely to have spontaneous abortions or stillborn children if they inhale these gases at work.

The table also lists carcinogens (cancer-causing substances) as potential mutagens. There is a great deal of scientific evidence indicating that most substances which cause mutations (especially in test-bacterial systems) are also capable of causing cancer. However, since it has not been definitely established that either this or the reverse case is always true, the table takes a conservative approach, and the carcinogens are also listed. Further, because there should be no unnecessary exposure to carcinogens for any worker—pregnant or not, male or female—contact with them, even if some are not found to cause mutation, should be absolutely avoided on the basis of cancer danger to the present generation.

An examination of the chemicals and exposures listed in the table reveals that a wide range of hazards exists for a large number of occupations filled by women workers. Hospital and health-care workers, flight attendants, various industrial workers, retail clerks, even teachers, all have potential exposure to reproductive hazards.

Non-occupational Environmental Defects

Workplace conditions are by no means the only villains causing birth defects, unsuccessful pregnancies, or other problems associated with childbearing.

Cigarette Smoking

Cigarette smoking is considered by many, the author included, to be the number one public-health hazard in the United States. About one third of all American women of childbearing age are smokers, and about 20–25 percent smoke during pregnancy.

Every scientific study on the effects of smoking during pregnancy has shown that smokers produce smaller babies than nonsmokers do. Figure 27 is a graph of the percentage of babies born over a given weight range to smokers and nonsmokers. The smokers' curve is shifted to the left, mean-

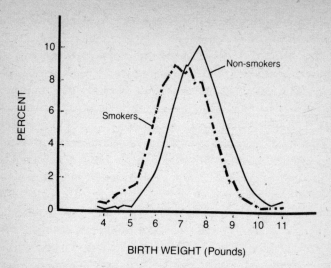

Figure 27. MOTHER'S SMOKING AND INFANT WEIGHT
The dotted line shows the lower weight distribution of infants
whose mothers smoked at least one pack of cigarettes per day in
comparison to the infants of nonsmoking mothers, represented
by the solid line.

SOURCE: U. S. Department of Health, Education and Welfare. *Health
Consequences of Smoking* (Washington, D. C., 1976), p. 419.

ing that the average birth weight of smokers' offspring is
lower than that of nonsmokers' offspring. There are more
small babies and fewer large ones.

The birth weight of an infant is related to its survival
rate, and studies of fetal and newborn deaths have indicated
an increased risk for the offspring of smokers. Both for birth
weight and for mortality there is a dose-response relationship, which means that the degree of the effect is related
to the number of cigarettes smoked: the more cigarettes,
the lower the birth weight. It is important to understand
that risk means probability, not certainty. All cigarette
smokers will not have small-for-date children; they just will
have a greater chance of bearing them than will nonsmokers.

Oxygen is essential for normal growth and development.
The presence in the blood of carbon monoxide, a major

component of cigarette smoke, very effectively deprives the body of oxygen. Again, a dose-response relationship has been demonstrated for carbon-monoxide levels: the more cigarettes smoked, the higher the carbon-monoxide blood level. The blood of a newborn of a smoking mother contains about a 9 percent carbon-monoxide level, which in effect decreases the amount of oxygen available. The percentage decrease corresponds to about a 41 percent blood-flow decrease. The blood samples in this study were taken after labor and are probably an underestimate, since most women do not smoke during labor, and the carbon-monoxide level drops rapidly when smoking ceases.[5]

Several other facts related to smoking have been discovered. The elements of cigarette "tar" (e.g., polycyclic aromatic hydrocarbons), which are associated with cancer, cross the placenta and enter the fetal bloodstream. There is also a decrease in vitamin C and vitamin B_{12} in the fetuses of smokers. The significance of these facts is not yet known.

While workplace environmental effects may be beyond a woman's control, smoking is not; and it must be obvious that women should stop smoking during pregnancy.

Drugs

The effects of several drugs taken during pregnancy and pregnancy outcome are given in Table 23. The best policy, and the one that most physicians adopt, is that no medicine is the best medicine during pregnancy. Of course, there may be situations in which some medication is necessary, and then a physician should choose it carefully. A woman should not hesitate to ask her physician whether a drug is really necessary and what its human effects are during pregnancy. She should specifically request to see the manufacturer's recommendation. If she feels that her doctor is not prudent or not open with her, it may not be a bad idea for her to find another physician more to her liking and more cognizant of her intellectual abilities.

TABLE 23. DRUGS AND PREGNANCY

The effect that a drug may have on the outcome of pregnancy will depend on the time that the drug is taken, the amount, and the length of exposure. For some drugs there may be differences in susceptibility.

DRUG	ASSOCIATED DEFECTS
Alcohol	Abnormally small head (microcephaly), eyelid abnormalities; possible heart, joint, and genital defects.

Steroid Hormones
  birth control pills
  androgens and progestins (male hormone)
 	
  DES
	All estrogen (female) hormones given early can induce abortion; given late, can become transplacental carcinogens. Inadvertant administration early in pregnancy associated with abnormality of spine, anus, windpipe, heart, and limbs. DES has been found to increase cervical cancer in female offspring and genital abnormalities in males.

Barbiturates
  Anticonvulsants
  Dilantin
  Phenobarbital
  Primidone
	Associated with head and face abnormalities.

Chemotherapeutic Agents
  Aminopterin
  Chlorambucil
  Cyclophosphamide
  Methotrexate
  Mitomycin-C
	Used in treatment of cancer patients, these agents cause serious damage to the embryo and may result in either death or severe deformation.

Thalidomide	When taken between the twentieth and thirty-fifth day, results in gross abnormalities of the musculo-skeletal system, such as defect in development of arms and legs.
Hypoglycemic Drugs Insulin	High incidence of dead or malformed fetuses found in women given high doses during insulin coma. Adverse effects of insulin maintenance not recorded.
Tolbutamide	About 1 out of 20 women maintained on this drug have been found to give birth to malformed infants, but this result is not universally accepted. Highly teratogenic in test animals.
Salicylates Aspirin	No known cases of gross defects in humans, but rats and monkeys have produced deformed fetuses. When combined with benzoic acid, a widely used food preservative, there is a

greater incidence in monkeys. Has been associated with impairment of blood-clotting factor (decreased platelet aggregation).

Antibiotics
  Streptomycin
  Tetracycline
  Others that cause
     defects in animals:
  Milomycin-C
  Actinomycin-D
  Penicillin-Streptomycin
     combination
	Not all antibiotics cause birth defects. If a woman needs antibiotic therapy and even suspects she is pregnant, she should inform her physician. Have been associated with deafness in offspring. Can lead to yellowing of first teeth.

A tragic example of drug use during pregnancy is the effect of the synthetic female hormone diethylstilbesterol (DES), which was administered to thousands of women in an attempt to prevent miscarriage. Although defects were induced in animals given DES, the drug was still used and approved for humans. It has now been shown that the teen-age girls and young women offspring of women given the drug have a high risk of developing cancer of the cervix. This is an instance of what is known as transplacental carcinogenesis, which means induction of cancer by substances crossing the placenta and affecting the developing fetus. Cancer of the cervix is virtually never found in women of this age group. DES and other hormones can cause a new-born female to develop masculine characteristics as well.

Male offspring of women to whom DES was administered have been found to develop abnormalities of the genital tract; they have not developed cancer as yet.

High levels of DES have been found in drug-manufacturing facilities that produce this hormone. No one knows what the results of inhaling DES during pregnancy are, but it is surely a situation which should be investigated.

Breast-feeding

Women who choose to breast-feed their babies should be aware that substances in the mother's bloodstream can pass into her milk supply. If she is exposed to fumes of heavy metals, such as lead, mercury, or cadmium, or if she uses or works with pesticides, which can be inhaled or absorbed through the skin, these will enter the milk. Women in Michigan who ate foods contaminated with the chemical PBB were found to have measurable levels of PBB in their milk. The same is true for drugs. Although toxic substances have a different effect when they enter the bloodstream through the digestive system than when they are inhaled, they can still be quite dangerous. Lactating (nursing) mothers should be conscious of these sources of potential hazards. Many state or city health departments will test breast milk for contaminants.

Likewise, cigarette smoking will result in nicotine entering the milk. Cases have been reported in which excess nicotine has caused diarrhea, vomiting, restlessness, abnormal heartbeat, and other symptoms of nicotine poisoning in the nursed newborn. Long-range lower-dose effects are unstudied.

There is also the possibility that stress and adverse working conditions can affect the mother's ability to produce an adequate milk supply.

Effects on the Mother

Pregnancy involves many maternal biological changes. Some of them are obvious; for instance, pregnant women carry around a great deal more body weight than do nonpregnant women. Other changes, such as chemical alterations of the blood, are more subtle and still not well understood. Two major body systems that are modified and that will be discussed here are the circulatory system and the respiratory system.

The circulatory system functions as a transit system for the body by transporting blood through the blood vessels. Blood carries oxygen to the various organs; transports toxic chemicals to the liver to be detoxified; and brings carbon dioxide, a waste product, to the lungs to be removed. During pregnancy, the volume of blood increases to accommodate metabolic and oxygen needs of the developing fetus, as well as to transport fetal waste products. Total blood volume increases by about 30–40 percent, reaching a maximum at about the thirty-fourth week of pregnancy and plateauing there until after birth. In addition, the veins in the uterus and in the lower part of a woman's body expand greatly during pregnancy. Additional blood is needed to fill up the increased volume so that there will be a steady flow of blood and oxygen to the mother's heart, brain, and other organs.

The increased blood volume adds to the work load of the heart as it pumps the blood. In addition, as pregnancy progresses, the uterus grows heavier and heavier, obstructing circulation by pressing on major blood vessels. As a result of the expanded leg veins, blood tends to form pools in the lower extremities, much the same way it does after one has been sitting, feet on the ground, in one position, for a long time. Blood pooling is especially noticeable if the woman lies flat on her back, a posture in which the uterus most effectively blocks circulation. Problems in circulation can be partially overcome by movement, elevating the legs, and so on. Obviously, jobs that require many hours of sitting in one position without adequate time and space for movement can be uncomfortable or even difficult, and it is useful to remember that such jobs are not conducive to good health at any time.

A pregnant woman also needs about 20–30 percent more oxygen than usual in order to keep her own enlarged body and that of the fetus functioning; consequently, her breathing patterns change. Although the total amount of air that she breathes (the vital capacity) does not change in itself, the rate and volume of breathing increases, as does the amount of air that is exhaled. Less reserve air remains in the lung after each exhalation, and the lung is relatively more collapsed. An increase in exhaled volume (technically known as tidal volume) increases lung efficiency in mixing gases in the air, since there is less air left in the lungs to dilute the new air breathed in.

It is difficult to make generalizations about the effects of changes in circulation or respiration on the ability to perform work. This is evidenced by scientific studies on exercise and pregnancy, which indicate that each woman's ability to exercise or do strenuous work is really an individual matter, and that this ability may be limited, especially as the pregnancy advances. If a woman has options available, she will generally try to restrict her activity to meet her physical needs. But if she has children to care for, a job with inadequate maternity provisions, housework, and so on, her only alternative will be to pace herself as best she can.

Modifications in the respiration rate and reserve air in the lung may be a hazard for the pregnant woman if she is working with toxic substances. Since her lungs mix gases more efficiently, those chemicals will enter her system more easily as well. The rate at which various chemicals are absorbed through the lungs is a function of how well the chemical dissolves in the blood, as it is the blood that transports gases which enter the lungs. A pregnant woman's blood contains different percentages of many normal constituents. It is unclear how this affects gas absorption. There is no real understanding yet of whether the response of the pregnant woman to toxic gases is different from that of the nonpregnant woman. This lack of knowledge is a reflection of the paucity of research on women's occupational health problems combined with a focus on fetal rather than maternal effects.

It is reasonable to assume, however, that there may be an

increased toxic effect in some cases, especially since the increased output of the heart causes more blood to come into contact with the gases efficiently.

During pregnancy, there is an increased production of blood components, particularly red blood cells. These contain hemoglobin, a large iron-containing molecule, which serves the function of transporting oxygen. Each hemoglobin molecule contains four atoms of iron, each of which can hold a molecule of oxygen until it reaches an organ or a part of the body that is oxygen-deficient. It then releases the oxygen and becomes available for transporting carbon dioxide to the lungs, where it will be exhaled. Ranges for the amount of iron in the blood of a normal female have been developed; and a deficiency of iron is called anemia.

Many pregnant women have been told that they are anemic, a state often called the physiological anemia of pregnancy. What actually happens in pregnancy is that the increased blood volume decreases the concentration or relative percentage of iron in the blood, bringing it below the normal levels of the nonpregnant state. There is no disease associated with this "anemia." In fact, it is the normal state for pregnant women, except in very rare cases. But the question of a decreased percentage of hemoglobin may be relevant for women who are exposed to lead, benzene, X-irradiation, and other conditions that also affect the body's ability to produce red blood cells normally. Although such exposures are dangerous for all workers, and pregnant women in particular, no definitive research has yet been done. However, some of the fetal effects are known and have been listed previously.

As we have seen, the heart is affected by environmental and emotional stress. The stress response (see Chapter Two) is the body's biological reaction to a stressful input. Emotionally stressful conditions, as well as physically stressful ones, can cause the release of chemicals that make the heart beat more rapidly and the blood pressure rise. Since the heart already has the increased burden of pumping more blood through expanded blood vessels, stress can only increase its work further. Thus, during pregnancy, as well as at other times, stressful working conditions can and do adversely affect health.

The physiological changes that accompany pregnancy are summarized in Table 24 along with aspects of employment that may be troublesome or perhaps dangerous to a woman during pregnancy and maternity.

The Role of the Male in Reproduction

Another aspect of the successful outcome of a pregnancy is the role of the father in determining the health of the offspring. Half the genetic material that makes up the fertilized egg comes from the male sperm. There is no reason to doubt that substances which can cause mutations in female sex cells can also cause mutations in those of the male. For instance, X-rays are known to cause chromosomal defects in males as well as in females, and chromosomal analyses of males working with various chemicals have also demonstrated that abnormal changes occur.

Many times the effect of workplace hazards on male genes is overlooked. We have almost come full circle from the belief held only a few hundred years ago that woman's function was simply to serve as a vessel for the father's offspring, to the present stance, wherein only the woman is denied employment and opportunity in order to prevent potentially adverse effects on the baby, while the vulnerable male suffers no such stigma.

Exposure to toxic chemicals and adverse working conditions can also affect the male's ability to successfully produce and implant sperm. Impotence or insufficient numbers of sperm or sperm that do not move effectively enough to fertilize the egg can arise from workplace hazards.

TABLE 24. REPRODUCTIVE HAZARDS OF WORK: MOTHER

The first column shows major biological changes of pregnancy. Also listed are some chemical conditions and occupations associated with possible adverse effects on these systems. Occupations which employ relatively few women are not listed even if they involve exposures to these substances. The table is not complete. More information can be obtained from the references listed in the Bibliography.

BODY SYSTEM	POTENTIAL HAZARDS	SOME OCCUPATIONS WHERE MIGHT BE FOUND
Lungs: Air is breathed more deeply, mixed more efficiently. There may be more effective absorption of toxic materials and deeper penetration of harmful dusts.	Toxic gases, fumes, and vapors Dusts	Agricultural workers Bookbinders Dental technicians, dentists Dry cleaners Electrical-parts workers Hairdressers and cosmetologists Lab technicians Meat wrappers Operating-room personnel Postal workers Sewers and stitchers Textile workers
Blood: Reduced percentage of hemoglobin and iron. There may be an enhanced effect of oxygen-depriving toxic chemicals and conditions.	Solvents—particularly benzene and other aromatics Chlorinated hydrocarbons (e.g., carbon tetrachloride, vinyl chloride, chloroprene) Carbon monoxide Aniline dyes and nitro compounds (methemoglobinemia formers)	Agricultural workers Bookbinders Cosmetics- and drug-manufacturing workers Dye workers Electrical-parts workers Hairdressers and cosmetologists

[171]

TABLE 24. (*Continued*)

BODY SYSTEM	POTENTIAL HAZARDS	SOME OCCUPATIONS WHERE MIGHT BE FOUND
	Amines and nitrates Metals (e.g, lead, nickel, cadmium) Pesticides (particularly chlorinated hydrocarbons)	Laboratory workers Lead-battery workers Packers and canners Rubber workers
Circulatory system: 30–40 percent greater blood volume; expanded blood vessels in legs and uterus; increased heart output; increased body weight. There may be a greater effect from jobs involving physical exertion or lack of it.	Standing or sitting too long Too strenuous activity Unreasonable lifting and carrying Stress (including noise and heat stress) Nitrates and other chemicals which affect circulation and heart function Rotating shifts	Agricultural workers Assembly-line workers Hotel workers Laboratory workers Laundry workers Nurses and nurses' aides Office workers Postal workers Retail clerks Service workers: cleaning and caretaking

Unfortunately, there is no extensive body of knowledge available in this area either. Table 25 summarizes much of what is known about the effects of working conditions on male reproductive abilities.

TABLE 25. EFFECTS OF SELECTED OCCUPATIONAL HEALTH HAZARDS ON MALE REPRODUCTION

Those agents which have been found to have adverse effects on male reproduction are listed. There has not been extensive research in the area.

AGENT	EFFECT
Benzene	Exposed workers found to have significantly higher chromosomal aberrations. Possible genetic effects on offspring.
Cadmium	Cadmium chloride can induce severe damage to testicular tissue and permanent sterility in test animals. Damage to the blood system of the testes and other parts of the male reproductive organs has also been observed in humans.
Lead	Low levels of lead have been reported to interfere with spermatogenesis in humans, yielding low sperm counts.
Manganese	Impotence and a decrease in libido have been reported.
Kepone	A high percentage of kepone-exposed workers suffered sterility.
Deuterium oxide	Mice exposed to this substance have become sterile. No results from human studies reported.
Radiation X-rays	Male radiological technicians in Japan found to have elevated incidence of sterility. Ionizing radiation also associated with chromosomal aberrations.
Gamma rays	Sterility in mice has been induced by gamma-ray exposure.
Excessive heat	Elevated temperature adversely affects male fertility.

At the time of printing, another chemical, a pesticide known as DBCP, has been implicated as causing sterility in male workers. However, several companies have not officially confirmed this because they now "suspect" that other antifertility agents may be present, such as ethylene dibromide and ethylene oxide, two substances not previously related.

CHAPTER FIVE

SOCIAL DISEASES . . . SOCIAL CURES

INDUSTRIALIZATION and urbanization have changed the fundamentals of human existence. The workplace has been wrest from the home, and a division of labor within the family has been created: homemaking and family care are quite different now from economically productive work outside the home. Since nature defines women as the child-bearers, and since the patterns of industrialization have not accommodated the patterns of childbearing and nurturing, a woman's ability to participate continuously in external marketplace activities is limited if she bears children. This places her in a distinctly disadvantageous position.

The economic disadvantages for women when work demands their presence away from home are not new. Historian Elise Boulding has described the effects of familial constraints on women wage laborers as early as the Middle Ages:

> Because of their immobility women have no bargaining power and so suffer wage discrimination everywhere. In 1422 the scholars of Toulouse paid women grape pickers

half what they paid the men, who only had to carry the full baskets back to the college cellar. (The monks of Paris did the same.) Women construction workers who worked side by side with men in building the College of Toulouse were paid far less than the men for the same labor.[1]

Of course, women in the Middle Ages who sold their labor away from home were the exception, because society was still largely rural and agrarian. But the home and child constraints on outside employment for women were apparently little different in their effect then than now.

Sexual role assignments do not correspond to reality. For example, 7.2 million women who were heads of households and supported their families in 1975, women without families, men with families and no wives, unmarried men— millions of American adults—do not fit into the accepted stereotype and hence suffer economically and socially by being required to provide all the aspects of the division of family labor for themselves. While some women, in fact, have remained in the home, raising children and running household affairs, a significant percentage of women, as we have seen, have never participated in childbearing. Even greater numbers of women have combined all three functions: workplace activity, home management, and childbearing and raising.

Further, we have seen that the conception of women as homemakers and childbearers and not as workers has affected many aspects of women, their work, and their health. Stress on the job and from the dual role of worker and homemaker, unrecognized and unstudied occupational health hazards, potential reproductive hazards, and the lack of a coherent social structure to aid women in their multifaceted obligations are but some of the results of mythologizing the status of women.

Perils of Protection

Industrialization, of course, affected more than the economic lives and roles of women. The early Industrial Revolution was marked by conditions that robbed life of its beauty, people of their health, children of their youth, and the environment of its natural goodness. Books like Dickens's *Hard Times* and Sinclair's *Jungle* amply illustrate the horrors of unfettered industrialism. The middle class, which ran the factories and offices, suffered along with the working class, which populated them, although not to the same physical degree. Stresses and pressures of the intense competition began to take their toll on the men, and the women were forced into the empty Victorian mold of the leisured woman. Weakness, silliness, and illness became their lot.

We have already discussed the peculiar role played by women and children in ameliorating the conditions of the early factories. Establishing protections for women was a driving wedge toward establishing these same rights—a minimum wage, an eight-hour day, and overtime pay—for all working people. We have also already noted that the advances first secured by women workers were generally granted on the basis of sexist generalizations about the "weaker" sex and the need to preserve the health of women in order to "preserve the species" rather than on the basis of human rights. Further, not all protective legislation benefited women workers or were extended to men. A series of restrictive regulations were passed by most states, curtailing the night hours that a woman could work or the maximum weight that she could lift. Often these regulations specified conditions far less rigorous than the daily chores most women carried out in their homes.

The legislation is even more contradictory because with hardly an exception, the restrictions against lifting heavy weights and night hours of work excluded coverage for those very jobs in which women were essential and needed protection. Hospital workers were permitted to work at night, and waitresses were allowed to lift heavy trays. Jobs in which women could earn more money or work their way up the social ladder, however, were often closed to them by the strict application of restrictive legislation. The justification for these laws was that they protected the health of women workers, but the laws were colored by a hypocrisy that casts this rationale into question.

So women were caught in a paradoxical situation. On the one hand, the rights that they gained, like the eight-hour day, were beneficial for all workers; on the other hand, other restrictions on weight lifting and night work would have been beneficial to all workers if extended to men, but they weren't. Thus, the protections that women "won" placed them in second-class economic roles. Although Title VII of the Civil Rights Act has struck down those state protective laws that result in discrimination in employment opportunity, a new era of protectionism for women workers seems to be surfacing. Faced with a variety of chemical and physical hazards in the workplace, modern lawmakers and policy makers have been pondering the "problem" of the exposure of women of childbearing capacity to such substances. What, if any, they ask, is the effect of such exposure on reproductive ability? Can exposure be prevented? How susceptible are the embryo and fetus to these hazards? The ability to answer these questions is limited, as we have seen throughout this book. Despite this, safety and health standards, disallowing the employment of fertile women, are now being proposed.

Further, health hazards on the job, such as stress and exposure to toxic chemicals, are usually perceived as having a different impact on women than on men. Women are inevitably categorized as childbearers whose contributions as workers are ancillary to the economy, and men as the main workers are breadwinners. One result is that the general health effects of dangerous chemicals or adverse working conditions are studied and regulated for male workers, and conditions that may adversely affect reproductive health are studied and regulated for female workers.

The Ironies of Lead

It is ironic that the best illustrations for the sexual misconceptions of occupational health are policies and standards for exposure to lead dust. As we shall see, the misrepresentations and fallacies about the greater effects of lead on women and childbearing have been circulating so long that by now they should be banal and trite. Instead, it has become a general policy of the Lead Industries Association, Inc., for example, that "no fertile, gravid [pregnant] or lactating female be employed in the lead industries until such time as adequate information has been developed regarding the effect of lead. . . ."[2] That policy has already been enacted by several large companies, and fertile women have been displaced from their jobs.

This policy is merely a restatement of old hiring practices only temporarily, it seems, set aside by Title VII. Because in the past women have been barred from lead exposure in heavy industry (but, of course, not in lower-paying industries, like pottery work, where there is also lead exposure), the actual numbers of women affected directly by such an exclusionary policy are small; however, the numbers would be enormous were this policy extended to other industries with other potentially toxic exposures.

The case is even more ironic when we consider that lead poisoning has been known as an occupational health hazard since ancient times, when lead miners were recognized to have the disease. That a modern society should still be seeking to "protect" unborn children while allowing other adults to be endangered by this ancient poison is the ultimate irony.

A proposal like the Lead Industries' policy to bar fertile

women from working with lead is very revealing. It recon-
firms the bias that continually surrounds women workers.
Just because a woman *can* bear children, it is presumed that
she *will* bear children—the perpetual pregnancy myth. And,
of course, the proposed standard implicitly presumes that a
woman cannot *choose* whether to continue to work in a
particular workplace once she is apprised of the potential
risks. The standard removes from the woman the ability to
choose: it mandates what is good for her and her offspring.

There are other more subtle dangers in the proposal. As
just noted, the exclusionary policy implies that barring
women solves the lead-exposure problem for workers. It
doesn't. Lead is harmful to all people, especially to children.
It affects the body's ability to produce red blood cells; it
can damage the nervous system; and it has been related to
kidney disease and high blood pressure, as well as other
adverse effects. Despite this, a proposed federal standard for
occupational exposure to lead would permit blood lead
levels in workers that are 50 percent higher than the maximum safe levels recommended for adults by the United
States Public Health Service.

Further, there is good evidence that lead affects male
reproductive ability. Male lead workers have been found to
have abnormal sperm production when their blood contained comparatively low lead levels—lower than recommended Public Health Standards for adults. Also, because
lead dust can contaminate clothing and shoes, lead workers
can and do inadvertently bring lead into their homes.
Children of lead workers have been found to have excessively
high levels of lead in their blood.

Thus, barring women from lead exposure by not letting
them work in lead industries may neither safeguard human
reproduction nor prevent the children already born from
suffering the effects of lead. It will not prevent adverse effects
in adults. There seems to be an aura of sanctity about a
fertilized egg, a sort of fetus fetish, that apparently disap-

pears when a child is born or matures into a working person. How else can one explain a health standard that ostensibly seeks to keep a fetus healthy but allows children and adults to be exposed to known harmful levels of lead?

There is one partial explanation. Coalition of Labor Union Women (CLUW) President Olga Madar stated it in her testimony on the lead standard proposed by the Occupational Safety and Health Administration.

> Industry's worry about harm to a fetus stems not from humanitarianism, but from fear that the fetus may be born deformed and live to sue them successfully for its injuries. As remote a possibility as that is, it weighs heavier on their minds than taking the steps necessary to prevent such harm to any of the offspring of either male or female workers by cleaning up the workplace.[3]

The testimony given by CLUW and other women's groups with respect to the proposed standard is reminiscent of the testimony given throughout the early industrial era by women's groups seeking to preserve the economic integrity of women in the face of restrictive legislation. History seems to be eternally repetitive.

A Study in Contrasts

Another irony is that while an exclusionary lead standard in itself may not endanger many women's jobs (since women in the past have systematically been excluded from higher-paying industrial jobs with lead), its ability to act as a precedent for excluding women from many other jobs, which present real or imagined adverse reproductive effects, is of staggering proportions. Because of the steadfast opposition of women's groups like CLUW, the National Organization for Women, Health-Right, and others, the proposed lead standard may be amended. It will certainly be contested in the judicial system if it is not amended. But far more fundamental changes in attitude and policies will be necessary to keep other "lead standards" from being promulgated.

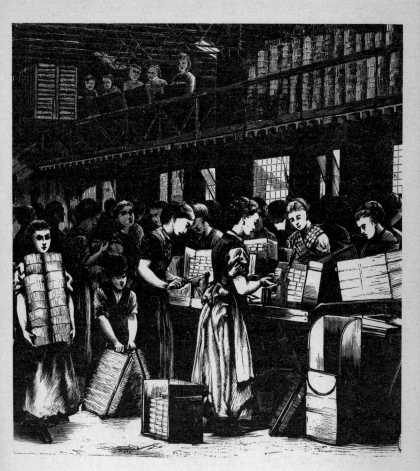

Illustration 2. WOMEN WORKERS MAKING MATCHES

These women workers making lucifer matches were exposed to phosphorus, which caused their jaws to erode, a condition called phossy jaws. This painful, disfiguring disease is the only occupational disease to have been completely eliminated. This was accomplished by various international laws and conventions early in the twentieth century which prohibit the manufacture of phosphorous matches.

SOURCE: *Harper's Weekly*, June 17, 1871.

It is interesting to contrast the government's position on lead to its position on the occupational exposure of pregnant women to ionizing radiation like X-rays. The National Commission on Radiation Protection (NCRP), responsible for formulating rules and regulations on radiation exposure, has issued guidelines for pregnant women working under this workplace hazard. These guidelines state that an employer must warn a woman of the potentially hazardous effects of radiation during pregnancy and must allow her the option of job transfer or temporary leave from her job, without penalty, if no transfer is possible.

The guidelines had originally mandated a limit for exposure to radiation for fetuses that was much more strict than the exposure limit for adult workers. In essence, this would have meant that there would be many workplaces, such as hospitals and dentists' offices, from which pregnant women would be excluded because working conditions would expose the fetus to radiation dosages that far exceeded the low fetal standard. However, because women are essential to health-care facilities, further consideration led the NCRP to change the mandated lower-dosage standards merely to the provision of warnings and information on options for voluntary job transfer or leave where no other job was available.

Of course, this is still not a viable solution to the basic dilemma. All living organisms are adversely affected by ionizing radiation, no matter how small the dose. Of course, the higher the dose, the greater the biological effect. Many experts feel that current workplace exposure standards are not really safe for the adult (see pages 100–2). The options in the guidelines may technically be open to a woman; but if her economic survival depends on a job that includes radiation exposure, does she really have an option if there is no job to which she can transfer? Further, because radiation can also affect a male's ability to reproduce successfully, the NCRP regulatory guidelines may actually discriminate against men, thereby continuing to fail to protect reproduction.

Again, history seems to be repeating itself. Protective laws that keep women from higher-paying jobs—like those in the lead industry—would safeguard women on the basis of reproductive health and allow men to be exposed to the dangers. On the other hand, jobs in health care, where women are essential, would once again be unregulated, despite potential consequences. The offhanded manner with which the government deems to give away women's jobs in heavy industry under the proposed lead standard is remarkably different from its attitude toward women working in the health industry, where their labor is essential. It is especially remarkable since ionizing radiation is *known* to be related to birth defects and abnormalities at levels below those considered safe for both male and female adults, while exposure to lead is *not known* to cause human defective births at levels below those which adversely affect the adult.

In addition, the data on male reproductivity and both ionizing radiation and lead exposure reveal that neither the radiation guidelines nor the proposed lead exposure standard is adequately protecting reproduction. We can also ask if it is discrimination against men to allow them to work under conditions that may adversely affect their health, while providing fertile women with protection from these conditions. Is it discrimination against all workers to consider hazards only in relation to their reproductive effects rather than in relation to their long-range health effects as occupationally hazardous conditions? It is clearly a serious dilemma when a worker must choose between a job, a livelihood, and the possibility of damage to oneself and one's unborn children. Yet, that is the only choice currently available in some situations.

The legal and moral aspects of the problem of reproductive hazards of work will not be easily resolved. The history of protective legislation is tinged with many similar political, social, and moral overtones. Certainly the problem is not new:

> The points to be considered for . . . a maternity policy are: the importance of judging each case individually, the time at which a woman should stop work before the birth of her child, and how soon afterward she may return to work; the types of jobs that should be avoided because of danger of physical strain or injury from toxic substances; the preservation of seniority rights, the opportunity to return to her job, the length of hours and rest periods, and other conditions of work.
>
> —1944, Women's Bureau[4]

Partial resolution can be expected through the courts, through legislation, and through union-management collective-bargaining agreements. But there will be no resolution unless the special needs of all workers are accounted for. Pregnant women, handicapped workers, older workers, semi-skilled workers, all need fair and equitable treatment, not merely exclusionary policies. And all workers need the guarantees of the Occupational Safety and Health Act of 1970 (OSHA), which provides that every man and woman is entitled to a workplace free from recognized hazards and that employers have the obligation of providing such a workplace.

The Law, Safety, and Health

Legal arguments can be made contesting the right of a company to transfer or fire women in order to purportedly safeguard their unborn, developing fetuses or, as the Lead Industries Association's policy implies, to safeguard their unconceived, perhaps never-to-be-born, potential fetuses, based on the Constitution, on Title VII of the Civil Rights Act, and on OSHA. Thus, the impact on women goes far beyond endangering higher-paying jobs in heavy industry.

If the legal battles are lost, then the very rights and guarantees of OSHA and Title VII will be seriously undermined.

Under OSHA, which is administered by the Department of Labor, standards for workplace exposure to toxic substances and conditions are to be formulated and enforced, and workplaces are to be investigated and inspected. OSHA also has the right to penalize employers that maintain workplaces found to be in violation of the provisions of the act. Workers have the right to request an inspection of their workplace and can remain anonymous if they so desire. OSHA also provides that no worker shall be discriminated against for exercising her or his rights under the act.

Unfortunately, the progress of OSHA has been slow and its guarantees for safety and health not met. The penalties for violations are minimal, generally averaging less than $30 per violation. The anti-discrimination clause is poorly enforced, and OSHA's initiative in enforcing the act is usually barely noticeable. A major part of the problem has been that the two Administrations during which OSHA came into existence were dedicated to its destruction. In fact, former President Gerald Ford had vowed to "throw OSHA into the ocean." This attitude, of course, makes it difficult for the OSHA staff to perform its functions. The Carter Administration has appointed a woman, Eula Bingham, as head of OSHA and has been emphasizing the enforcement of the health aspects of the act; but only time will tell if meaningful change will occur.

Other excellent references are available on the history and practices of OSHA, and on workers' rights under the law. Some of these are listed in the Bibliography. Our discussion here will deal with the impact of OSHA on women workers.

A purpose of the Occupational Safety and Health Act is to "assure insofar as practicable that no employee shall suffer diminished health, functional capacity or life expectancy as a result of his [or her] work experience." Yet, in its proposed regulation for occupational exposure to lead, OSHA has raised the possibility that all women of child-bearing age need "special" standards to protect them, and it has recommended a lead standard that will permit blood lead levels that exceed the safe level for children—and, one would presume, for fetuses. The proposed standard would thus permit lead exposures that may be unsafe for pregnant women, since high blood lead in the mother will be found in the fetus as well. Furthermore, OSHA has mandated pregnancy tests for female employees in its prepared standard—an incredible invasion of privacy. Since the ability to reproduce is clearly a functional capacity, it is difficult to reconcile the proposed standard with Title VII, which prohibits discrimination in the workplace and other federal guarantees.

It is interesting that in its proposed standard, OSHA has returned to the special-susceptibility-of-women argument. We have already seen that women, in fact, are generally healthier than men, live longer, and develop fewer chronic diseases. Yet the female susceptibility argument persists. In the case of lead, which can affect production of the red blood cells, the argument becomes insidious. Red blood cells contain hemoglobin, a large iron-bearing molecule. Women have lower hemoglobin levels than men. Some scientists like to perceive this normal difference as a "relative insufficiency of iron" among females.[5] The absurdity of this statement becomes apparent if we reverse it, saying that men have a relative excess or overabundance of iron—an obviously nonsensical statement. Somehow, the nonsense seems to be lost when the false generalizations are about women.

It makes good scientific sense to assume that females have enough hemoglobin for female functioning, and males have enough for male functioning. There is no justification for using male norms for females, and vice versa. Yet we are continually surrounded by such irrational reasoning. Television commercials blare the benefits of various iron potions at us. Take tonic because "women need extra iron." Why? To bring their level up to that of men? Unfortunately, such reasoning has effectively blocked women from employment with lead exposure throughout many European countries and played a part in the formulation of the proposed new standard.

Of course, the use of fallacious data or a biased perspective is not new, especially with regard to the effects of lead. In 1902, Dr. Thomas Oliver wrote that "females contract lead poisoning more readily, the symptoms are usually more acute, they suffer more severely and succumb to it more quickly than males."[5] Anna Baettjer, in her book in 1946, analyzed the data and arguments of Oliver and others, and concluded that "on the basis of the data quoted above, there appears to be no very convincing evidence that women are more susceptible to lead poisoning than men." She also noted that "for the most part, the theory that women are more susceptible than men to occupational disease has arisen by the repeated quoting in the literature of statements to the effect made by one or two industrial health authorities. In many cases the statements represented only a personal opinion."[7]

It should not be surprising that these same unfounded generalizations and poor studies are still being cited in the scientific literature. As recently as 1976 they were referred to uncritically in a review of the literature with regard to reproductive hazards of lead:

> Lead has been known to affect women during pregnancy for more than a century. Teratogenesis has been reported and documented by animal experimentation. In addition to lead's direct adverse effect on the course of pregnancy, it has an indirect effect by its toxic action on the male germ cell. There is evidence that women, particularly during specific periods, i.e., adolescence, pregnancy, etc., are more susceptible to toxic effects of lead. Oliver has noted that women are more susceptible to lead poisoning

between the ages of 18 and 23, and after shorter exposure. He noted that women poisoned by lead have a higher incidence of encephalopathy, and a lower incidence of paralysis and colic, than males.[8]

This paper, in turn, has been cited by others. Once a fallacious statement or idea makes its way into the scientific literature, it is apparently difficult to remove it, especially if that statement or idea fits in with many other preconceived and unfounded generalizations based on sexual stereotypes.

Only Men Are Created Equal

The inability to provide equitable treatment to women did not end with safety and health in the workplace. We should not forget that it was only a little more than two generations ago that women gained the right to vote and that today the Equal Rights Amendment to the Constitution is being fought. Further, during the past several years, a majority of the Justices of the United States Supreme Court again failed to recognize the social needs and rights of women as workers and childbearers and have jeopardized the legal advances made by women under Title VII of the Civil Rights Act, which prohibits discrimination in employment. They have reinforced many of the myths and practices that have for decades been plaguing women as workers and as mothers. This failure of the judicial system is very much a reflection of the failure of society as a whole to recognize and meet the social needs of women.

In 1898, suffragette Elizabeth Cady Stanton observed:

> To me there is no question as important as the emancipation of women from the dogmas of the past, political, religious and social. It struck me as very remarkable that abolitionists who felt so keenly, the wrongs of the slave, should be so oblivious to the equal wrongs of their own mothers, wives and sisters, when, according to the common law, both classes occupied a similar legal status.[9]

The Civil Rights Act of 1964 finally did legally link the two causes of civil rights for blacks and for women, since that act made illegal discrimination based on race, color, religion, sex, or national origin.

However, it is important to note that despite the fact that sex is included in the list of discrimination taboos, the civil and equal rights of women were not a major issue during the passage of the act. The massive *New York Times Index* for 1964, for example, records thousands of entries on civil rights for black Americans but only a handful on women's rights. Many observers have concluded that sex was appended onto the original Civil Rights Act as a joke. Modern civil rights advocates were no more cognizant of women's rights than their nineteenth-century counterparts.

For example, the illegitimacy of the concept "separate but equal" facilities was, of course, at the heart of much of the Civil Rights movement for black Americans during the 1960s. A class-action suit brought by the parents of Susan Vorchheimer on behalf of all girls denied admission to a Philadelphia city high school for academically gifted males was turned down by the U.S. Supreme Court. Philadelphia maintains a similar school for girls, which the Board of Education, and the Court, deems to be "separate but equal" to the boys' school for academic excellence.

The Supreme Court has thus chosen to allow "separate but equal" facilities when they are based on sex and to overlook the psychological subtleties of separate schools, which never really allow girls' schools to equal boys' schools. For instance, the valedictorian of an all-girls' school is not really considered as bright and competent as the valedictorian of a boys' school or of a co-educational facility—after all, she had to compete only with other females. The words of Elizabeth Cady Stanton still ring true.

The Fourteenth Amendment to the Constitution, passed after the Civil War, guarantees equal protection and due process to all citizens:

. . . (the) State shall not deprive a person of life, liberty, property, without *due process* of law; nor deny to any person within its jurisdiction the *equal protection* of the laws.

The Fifth Amendment provides for similar liberties under federal statutes.

The *Federal Reporter* noted that "the regulations which established admission requirements based on gender classification did not offend the equal protection clause"[10] by the Vorchheimer case. They may not offend the clause, but they certainly offend all women and the true cause of justice.

One meaning of the phrase "due process" is that rules and regulations which treat all people as part of a class or sex and not as individuals cannot be set. It is not due process, for example, for an individual to be denied an opportunity or benefit only because that person is black or is handicapped. Each person must be allowed to demonstrate his or her capabilities and needs individually, and not simply be lumped into a stereotype.

Similarly, the equal protection clause was meant to guarantee that Americans receive equal treatment before the law. In actuality, not until the second quarter of the twentieth century was such judicial interpretation applied; and in the 1950s and 1960s, great legal strides toward insuring legal guarantees continued to be made. Finally, in 1964, nearly a century after the original passage of the Fourteenth Amendment, the Supreme Court ruled that it was unconstitutional and a denial of equal protection for voting districts not to give all citizens equal representation. Women's rights, however, made no similar progress. In fact, as we have seen, many facets of equal protection under the law for women *still* have not been affirmed by the courts today.

A recent case, brought by Carolyn Aiello and thirty other women employees in the State of California, is also illustrative. The women were covered by an Unemployment Disability Fund to which they, like all the other employees,

TABLE 26. A QUICK GUIDE TO SOME LEGAL RIGHTS OF WOMEN WORKERS

U. S. CONSTITUTION	LEGISLATION	ADMINISTERING AGENCY
Amendments Article XIV: Section 1: "All persons born or naturalized in the United States and subject to the jurisdiction thereof, are citizens of the United States and of the State wherein they reside. No State shall make or enforce any law which shall abridge the privilege or immunities of citizens of the United States; nor shall any State deprive any persons of life, liberty or property without the *due process* of law; nor deny to any person within its jurisdiction the *equal protection* of the laws." [Italics supplied by author.] (The Fifth Amendment provides the same protections as regards the federal government.)	Civil Rights Act of 1964, Title VII: guarantees the rights to employment without sex, race, color, creed, religion, or national origin discrimination	Equal Employment Opportunity Commission (EEOC)
	Equal Employment Opportunity Act of 1972: amends and broadens Title VII	
	Fair Labor Standards Act (1938): establishes minimum wage, overtime, etc.	Wage and Hour Division, Department of Labor
	Equal Pay Act (1963): last amendment to Fair Labor Standard Act	
	Occupational Safety and Health Act (1970): guarantees a safe and healthful workplace to all workers	Occupational Safety and Health Administration (OSHA), Department of Labor
	State FEP	Appropriate state agency

NOTE: There are separate bills and executive orders establishing coverage for federal employees for the provisions of these laws. Most states have also adopted such coverage for their state and local workers as well.

made regular contributions. During their pregnancies, they requested reimbursement from the fund for the time that they were unable to work; that is, they requested the same coverage as other workers who were temporarily disabled from work. They were denied such payments because of the language of the statutes.

Suit was brought against the state by the women on the basis that they were denied their Constitutional right to equal protection under the law. They argued that women, who were members of one sex, alone had the burden of bearing children; thus, denial of temporary work-disability coverage for pregnancy-related work disability had a clear, unequal, and disparate impact on them.

As a counterexample, their suit argued that men were covered by the fund for temporary work disabilities related to medical procedures, such as the removal of a prostate gland, which only men can undergo. Even work disability due to voluntary medical procedures, such as cosmetic surgery (e.g., face-lifts), were compensated, so that the dubious argument that pregnancy was a "voluntary" condition was not even justifiable.

Equal protection, the Court held, did not force the state to provide extensive social welfare programs. The Court further held that the state had a legitimate interest in maintaining the financial integrity of the disability fund, which, the Court concluded, might be jeopardized by including coverage for normal pregnancy-related work disability.

Justices Brennan, Douglas, and Marshall dissented. They wrote that the majority Court ruling was clear sex discrimination because:

1. disabilities suffered only by men or ethnic minorities were not excluded by the fund;

2. the adverse economic effects of employment disability, for which the fund had been designed, which were caused by pregnancy, were indistinguishable from other effects;

3. the increased cost was shown to be reasonable and could be met without undue hardship.

The dissenting opinion predicted that the decision "threatened to return men and women to a time when 'traditional' equal protection analysis sustained legislative classifications that treated differently members of a particular sex solely because of their sex." Since the Aiello Supreme Court decision, the State of California has enacted legislation which provides that work disabilities resulting from normal pregnancies are to be compensated for up to six weeks, and the statute now covers complications of pregnancy without limitations. Although such legislation tempers the immediate impact of the Supreme Court decision, it does not temper the prevailing attitude of the Court.

Legal Perils of Pregnancy

The Aiello case was tested and lost in the courts, using arguments based on the Fourteenth Amendment to the Constitution. However, other legal avenues, such as Title VII of the Civil Rights Act, which explicitly prohibits discrimination in employment practices, are available. The Equal Employment Opportunity Commission (EEOC) administers Title VII and is empowered to investigate complaints, to issue cease and desist orders to employers, and to issue decisions. However, enforcement is through the judiciary system, where the EEOC can sue in its own name and in the name of the complainant. The EEOC has issued guidelines, summarized in Table 27. However, despite these powers, dependence on the judiciary has resulted in a current case backlog, which is overwhelming. Several years will elapse before a woman will have her day in court, if she has the money, ability, and knowledge to pursue her case— and then her day may not turn out well.

For example, the EEOC guidelines are clear: for the purposes of all job-related benefits, pregnancy and maternity are

TABLE 27. A SUMMARY OF EQUAL EMPLOYMENT OPPORTUNITY COMMISSION SEX DISCRIMINATION GUIDELINES

Principles of equal employment opportunities apply to employers, labor organizations, and employment agencies. Title VII of the Civil Rights Act of 1964 (amended by the Equal Employment Opportunity Act of 1972) provides that no one shall be discriminated against on the basis of sex, race, color, or national origin in the area of employment.

Bona Fide Occupational Qualification (BFOQ): It is discriminatory to 1) label jobs as men's jobs or women's jobs; 2) refuse to hire a person because of stereotypes, like females lack sales aggressiveness or males do not have nimble fingers; 3) have state laws which (a) limit working for only one sex (e.g., weight-lifting limits and night-work restrictions) and do not take individual differences into account; (b) provide minimum wage and overtime only for females; (c) provide special rest facilities or meal requirements for one sex, thereby limiting employment opportunity for that sex and denying equal benefits to the other.

Separate seniority and progression lines based on sex unless there is a bona fide occupational qualification are illegal.

Discrimination against married women is illegal unless based on a bona fide occupational qualification.

Job opportunities advertising cannot be based on sex. Classified ad headings "male" and "female" are illegal.

Employment agencies must be aware of current EEOC guidelines, will share responsibilities with employers for discrimination, and cannot deal solely with one sex unless there is a bona fide occupational qualification.

Fringe benefits (pensions, profit sharing, insurance, etc.): 1) cannot discriminate between men and women (e.g., headings like "head of household" and "principal wage earner" tend to refer to men and cannot be used to define eligibility for benefits; 2) if wives of male employees are eligible for benefits, then so are female employees; 3) discriminatory practices cannot be defended on the basis of excess cost of coverage for one sex versus another; 4) separate requirements, such as retirement dates or separate benefit tables based on sex, are illegal.

*Pregnancy and childbirth**: 1) employment practices or policies based on pregnancy are illegal; 2) pregnancy is a temporary disability, like a broken leg or industrial accident, and shall be treated as such with respect to company practices for seniority, health insurance, etc.; 3) if there is no temporary disability policy and an employee is terminated because of a temporary disability like pregnancy, that termination is illegal if it has a special impact on one sex and cannot be justified by business necessity.

* See text, pages 195–7 for Supreme Court decision concerning this guideline.

to be considered temporary disabilities. This is not to say that under the EEOC guidelines, pregnant women or new mothers are considered "sick," but that if a woman seeks time off from her job because of pregnancy-related reasons, she should receive the same rights and privileges that other temporarily *work*-disabled workers receive. Disability insurance, the right to retain seniority and return to the job, pension rights, and so on were to be afforded to pregnant women and new mothers in the same way as they would be afforded to a worker with a broken arm or injured hip. Further, the guidelines provide that if a company does not have a maternity policy or temporary disability plan, where leave without penalty is granted, such a policy should be adopted.

In the General Electric v. Gilbert case, known as the Gilbert decision, the U. S. Supreme Court delivered a severe setback to the guidelines' universal guarantee of pregnancy and maternity disability insurance benefits, holding that the guidelines "sharply conflict" with proper interpretation of sex discrimination under Title VII of the Civil Rights Act. The Supreme Court made its ruling in a suit originally brought against General Electric, charging the company with discrimination because of its failure to provide maternity disability benefits according to the EEOC guidelines, and had been upheld by the U. S. Court of Appeals, the second highest court in the United States. Further, similar suits had been upheld in several other Appeals Courts.

The dissenting argument of Justice Brennan, with concurrence of Justice Marshall, is important for our understanding of the social meaning of the decision. The Justice wrote that the exclusion of pregnancy benefits by General Electric is merely part of a long history of sex discrimination by the company. Further, the Justice ridiculed the contention of the majority of the Court that exclusion of pregnancy is not "sex-related," a contention which "offends common sense." Part of his view is summarized in the following excerpt:

> The policy formulations [temporary disability plans] are reasonable responses to the uniform testimony of governmental investigations which show that pregnancy exclusions built into disability programs both financially burden women workers and act to break down the continuity of the employment relationship, thereby exacerbating women's comparatively transient role in the labor force. . . . In dictating pregnancy coverage under Title VII, EEOC's Guideline merely settled upon a solution now accepted by every other Western industrial country. . . . I find it difficult to comprehend that such a construction can be anything but a "sufficiently reasonable" one to be "accepted by the reviewing courts."

Just as with the Aiello case, an opposition movement has quickly organized to change the statute and to amend Title VII to explicitly prohibit discrimination on the basis of pregnancy, childbirth, or related medical conditions. However, women have obviously suffered a severe legal setback in their quest for equal rights and equal opportunity as economically productive citizens.

Bearing the Burden . . .

As noted by Justice Brennan in his dissent in the Gilbert decision, the United States is the only industrialized country in the world with no universal legal and social provisions for maternity. (The rights of pregnant workers are still a matter for legal debate in the courts.) There are no nationwide social insurance systems to help with finances, medical care, or maternity benefits. There are insufficient child-care facilities. There are few sick-leave policies designed to help the working mother care for her sick children. There is little social or economic recognition of the housework performed by women not also elsewhere employed. (And the recent Court rulings we have discussed have removed much of the legal "incentive" for such recognition.)

Women who are employed outside the home and have families are on their own. Women who care for children and work in the home are on their own. This, perhaps, is the most contradictory aspect of the female role: the simultaneous social glorification of motherhood and childbearing, and the social unwillingness of men to aid women in fulfilling these roles. The same society that sings the praises of motherhood is strangely mute in helping mother keep home and hearth together.

Comparatively few women are able to escape from the various dilemmas of the dual role of home/family and work, which we have explored throughout this book. One illustration is a recent study of female physicians in Detroit. Physicians are the highest paid, most prestigious professionals in our society. Yet three out of four of the female physicians in the study saw to all their families' cooking, shopping, and child-care needs, in addition to attending to their patient-care duties. While they may have engaged outside help for some of these tasks, the responsibility of the work was still theirs.[11]

The female physicians earned less than the males and held less prestigious positions. (The study also found that their productivity remained high, despite the onerous double burden they carried.) In addition, it is interesting that about half of these women physicians (43 percent) were married to physicians. While in theory both marriage partners in such a situation could share many professional achievements *and* the responsibilities of the home, the study showed that home management and child-care were not shared; hence, the female physicians suffered professionally. This is especially interesting, since married physicians can choose specialties and adopt hours that could be complementary, in order to facilitate equitable work/home arrangements. Physicians who worked under such conditions would still earn far more money and achieve far more professional status than most other married couples could; and yet the study shows this did not happen. Obtaining a medical degree does not free a woman from her "female" role and her female "obligations," or even allow her to equitably share the work with her mate.

. . . Sharing the Burden

The crux of the problem is that although childbearing and nurturing are social functions, essential for the preservation of the human species, in the United States they are treated very much as an individual responsibility. The nuclear family, particularly the woman, is responsible for the basic needs of the children, and women who do not bear children, or have finished bearing children, are *assumed* to be childbearers, and they are thus kept in second-class economic roles.

Pregnancy, giving birth, and nurturing children are disruptive of the work norm of modern industrial society, where job advancement, security, training, and pensions all depend on unbroken years of work, which usually extends at least eight hours per day, over five days a week, and forty-eight to fifty weeks per year.

As we have already noted, such work patterns are universally difficult. The previous discussions of various aspects of stress amply illustrate that modern industrial practices and demands are intimately involved in the factors responsible for the toll of heart disease and other chronic illness in the United States today. Though the sources of stress for the two sexes are often quite different, stress itself is pandemic. Women with families suffer from an inability to conform to the modern industrial work norm, and men suffer from having conformed to the work norm for too long; families and children cannot escape the pressures either.

The years when parenthood is most demanding correspond to the years when job demands are most pressing. The most conscientious father usually cannot devote sufficient time to his family. Jobs with flexibility are few. Even university academic positions, possibly the most time-flexible jobs, require high productivity of young faculty members, who are generally the people with young families as well. If a woman can work only part-time, or not at all, during those high-productivity years, chances are that she will never be able to catch up.

The need for rapid occupational achievement is not confined to professional careers. Studies have found that a man who is not a foreman by his mid-thirties will probably never become one. The problem for women is obvious.

Men and women are both paying a price for the lack of a coherent, meaningful social policy toward parenthood and work. The constraints of our urban, industrial society, with its emphasis on individual social responsibility and high productivity, especially during one's twenties and thirties, are such that even if women and men were to exchange nurturing roles (the biological ones are immutable), it would simply be a rearrangement of social burdens, not an equalization of rights and privileges. Role exchange is not a solution.

"Making It"—The New Norm

The necessity for basic changes in the social system in order to afford more equitable treatment and opportunity for women, as well as others, is more urgent now than ever before, since we have entered an era that diverges so greatly from the Victorian era of the leisured woman, who was forbidden useful employment. The modern woman is quickly being forced into a new norm: the working woman. Magazines, newspapers, and television programs direct themselves to the new modern female.

Unfortunately, the rhetoric of the working woman has not been accompanied by the realities of a system geared to help women accomplish their tasks of working on the job and in the home, and raising a family. And the status of women on the job has not really improved either—despite the modern image. In a recent article, "Women and Power— A Status Report," *The New York Times* reported that "in the corporate world" there was "more talk than progress." Women still account for fewer than 1 percent of top management, and the all-important middle-management roles, which lead up the corporate ladder, have remained unchanged over the past two decades, at less than 6 percent female.[12]

In its analysis of why women are still not "making it," the *Times* cites such factors as ingrained prejudice among male executives, the fear of female competition, and the absence of a large pool of experienced women from whom to draw. These factors undoubtedly are important. But another major consideration as to why more women are not "making it" is that many women are unwilling to relinquish family and home life in order to climb the corporate ladders of success. Executive lives are demanding, and men do not have to make the choice. In fact, wife and family are almost essential to the successful corporate executive. A hard-working, ambitious executive female too often does have to choose. She doesn't have a wife at home.

The new norm is for women to work. The leisured woman of the Victorian era has been replaced by the married career woman of the twentieth century. And just as the social costs for women were great during the days of Queen Victoria, they remain great for the women of today. The problem is not to detail the ways in which women are "making it," but to figure out how they are going to combine home, family, and job, and love every minute of their eighty-hour week.

Some Modest Proposals

If women are to secure a place in the economy, and if the artificialities of the division of labor within the home created by industrialization and urbanization are to be eliminated, then societal accommodations to women's dual role of homemaker and worker are necessary. First, a re-evaluation of the economic value of homemaking and traditional fields of women's employment must be made. Next, specific programmatic innovations must occur in incentives for the employment of women; equal opportunity in training, job placement, and advancement; areas of hours of work; assistance in child-care; and ancillary changes in the tax structure to benefit working couples and single parents.

Social proposals and programs must, of course, be flexible and recognize individual choice. For some women, full-time work in the home may be a preferable alternative to part-time work at home and on the job. Others may opt for full-time employment throughout their working lifetimes, despite the responsibilities of home and family. Some couples may prefer to share household and economic responsibilities between the male and the female, others to reassign the traditional roles. The major point is that options and viable programs dealing with women's dual role must be made available.

It would be a useful social "rediscovery" to glance briefly at the mobilization of women workers that occurred during World War II. When it was essential to national survival to treat women as employable workers, child-care centers, flexible-shift jobs, and job sharing were among the social structures that appeared virtually overnight. After the war, they disappeared almost as quickly. Some suggestions for the partial resurrection of these abandoned programs follow.

The Work Norm

Although the structure of work as currently conceived requires forty hours per week of concentrated effort throughout one's working lifetime, many higher-paid and skilled jobs require mandatory overtime, and professional careers often demand an even greater time commitment. Social benefits, such as pensions, health insurance, and seniority rights, depend on unbroken years of workplace attendance. In licensed professions and crafts, failure to adhere to this work regime may result in loss of license; in other areas of work, it may make one's skills obsolete. The work norm often continues until retirement.

Parenthood, as well as a productive and healthy old age, is incompatible with the modern regime. Because the needs of young children do not adapt well to this work schedule, those women who must leave work for some time to raise families are clearly at a disadvantage. The rising incidence of stress-related chronic diseases seems to indicate that the middle-aged are not thriving, and the plight of the senior citizen, who is banished into debilitating retirement, and often into relative poverty, is well documented. Several alternatives, however, are available:

1. Flexible hours of work: If both men and women could work flexible hours, parents could coordinate household and child-care obligations, and a single parent could arrange hours to suit family needs. Flexible work hours do not necessarily imply continually changing hours; rather, they enable working people to select work schedules that accommodate family demands. Many industries could adapt to this type of work plan.

2. Part-time work: Jobs with flexible hours are usually full-time positions. However, both parents may not want a full-time job or may find it too difficult to manage one combined with the responsibilities of home and child care.

Currently, part-time jobs are often not well paying and do not lead to advancement and long-term security. A half-time job or a two-thirds-time job, which would allow one to accrue seniority and retain skills, especially during the years when home responsibilities are greatest, is an option that should be available for both men and women. Ancillary benefits, such as extended periods of time for attainment of tenure, permanent job status, professional experience, or whatever appropriate mark of progress or success each occupation has, are also necessary.

Child Care

Facilities and options for various child-care programs should be nationwide, subsidized and carefully supervised by trained personnel to assure quality care. The costs could be based on the ability to pay. Employers could contribute directly or into a fund similar to the social security system. The increased economic activity of working women would recompense for the investment.

Sick leave should be available to parents who must care for a sick child. In addition, a subsidized corps of trained health professionals should be created so that the sick child of a parent who must report to work can be left in the care of a responsible adult. Direct cost could again correspond to the ability to pay. Also, insurance plans could be extended to cover such at-home care.

Maternity and parenthood leaves must be options for the parent who desires to raise his or her child without the social and economic stigmas of losing job status and job opportunity. The years of intense child care are relatively short. For closely spaced children, this may mean that a parent could return to economic activity within as few as five or six years and still have given personal care to preschool children.

Economic Incentives

A national task force charged with the re-evaluation of the economic status of women's work at home and on the job should be created immediately, and its suggestions incorporated into a national economic program that could eliminate the poverty of large numbers of women and the economic exploitation of homemakers.

A national program for on-the-job training for women should be instituted, so that a woman with obsolete or irrelevant skills could be paid while learning. A job-acquirement program that truly offered equal opportunity and affirmative action is also necessary. In addition, a conscientiously directed national effort to redirect the interests and skills of women into economically viable channels is needed. Current practices destine women for women's work. The effort will have to begin as early as the preschool level, where many initial biases are instilled.

Of course, women will not succeed in gaining employment in diversified areas if other social programs, such as flexible work hours and child care, are not simultaneously adopted to accommodate the dual role of homemaker and worker. What is also needed is a full-employment economy, which would end the traditional marketplace position of the many women who have always served as an untapped surplus labor pool, thus depressing their market value.

Furthermore, the tax structure should be changed to benefit working people who are raising families, and a more realistic credit for child care should be provided. To end the tax bias against the working couple, it has been suggested that there could be a "general earned income credit, . . . but this creates a bias against investments in capital and in favor of wage income."[13] Such a bias could be helpful to women in their efforts to recapture their place in the economy.

Occupational Safety and Health

Health and safety standards must not exclude women from the workplace on the pretext of protecting the fetus from potential harm. However, standards must be stringent enough to protect adults, preserve their reproductive capability, and insure normal offspring. If sufficiently safe levels are not attainable, full transfer rights (e.g., retention of seniority, rate of pay, and the right to return to the original work) to less dangerous work must be afforded, since the embryo and fetus may be significantly more sensitive than the adult to the effects of certain conditions. If no such work can be found, then disability leave with pay must be provided. This must be available to those planning pregnancies and those in the early stages, for the embryo is most vulnerable at that time.

The disability payments could be provided by the individual employer, by an employee plan, by the federal government, or by a national health network.

Similar transfer rights must be available to potential fathers where their reproductive capabilities also could be compromised by their working conditions.

The Harsh Realities

The policies and realities of modern society obviously differ from the social programs and the goals of equality of treatment and opportunity outlined here. Current economic conditions make it unlikely that rapid change will occur. For so many women who are seeking to continue their education and re-enter the job market after bearing and raising children, the present deterioration of the economy has meant shorter library hours, higher tuition, less financial support, and less child-care aid. A library closed on Sundays may eliminate a mother's ability to use its facilities. A tuition raise may mean the choice between a woman's education and her family's needs. Most municipalities and school districts have been forced to cut back on after-school centers, school lunch programs, child-care centers, and other social-support systems, as limited as they are. These cutbacks may ultimately force a woman to leave her job in order to tend to her child during working hours.

Widespread unemployment and a recession have virtually eliminated flexible-shift experiments. Part-time work is also limited and has never been a meaningful stepping stone for advancement and job security. Another consequence of a sluggish economy has been massive layoffs and firings. Those who are the last hired are usually the first asked to leave. Too often these people will be women and minority workers who have finally managed to penetrate the barriers of discrimination. The question is whether society need choose between equality of opportunity and a worker's right to job security and seniority. A full-employment economy would surely end this dilemma.

In essence, the effect of the cutbacks serves to bring into focus the fundamental idea that to alter the condition of women, some of the basic practices of our society must be re-evaluated. The obligations of the social systems to the individual, and vice versa, are central to the matter. If women are to successfully fulfill their dual role of home-maker and worker, then a societal support structure incorporating some of the proposals mentioned here must be built to accommodate that dual role and to allow males to share it more fully. Childbearing and employment must be recognized as social rights and social functions for which social solutions must be provided. These solutions must allow fathers to participate in parenting as well. The elimination of prejudice and lack of opportunity for childbearing women will, of necessity, improve the lot of those women who are neither wives nor mothers but who have been burdened with the stereotypes that cast all women into the same die. Such social solutions will meld together the artificial triad—home, work, and family—that industrialization has created.

Is the System Working?

Fundamentally, we can ask the question of whether the social system is "working," not just for working women with families but for all individuals. Certainly the divorce rate, unemployment rate, poverty rate, delinquency rate, and crime rate are powerful testimony to the inability of our society to cope with its many social needs and social problems.

We can examine the isolated nuclear family, which too often keeps children from their grandparents, aunts, and uncles, and dissolves the familial support system that had been a part of human existence until urbanization and industrialization disrupted it. Each nuclear family is now forced to provide for itself all its survival needs, as well as housekeeping and child-care duties. The lack of success that this arrangement has had is evident from the 29 percent of all females who are divorced and from the fact that 13 percent of all families are headed by single women. The young are alienated; the middle-aged are striving and struggling toward heart disease, cancer, and the restlessness and uselessness of retirement; and the old are impoverished. The plight of women, their second-class citizenship, the dual-role dilemma, and perpetual mythologies are parts of the total problem.

Industrialized society must recognize that the components of the triad of daily existence—the job, the family, the home—do not really form a triad but are aspects of the wholeness and oneness of life. As long as the human right to a total existence is not recognized by modern society, women will not gain true equality but merely a more equal share of an unsatisfactory existence. The total liberation of women will occur when the workplace no longer offers hazards to any worker or to future generations, when the stress of job dissatisfaction and alienation is overcome, and when parents and children—and those people who do not become parents—are allowed to fully participate in social as well as economic roles for the betterment of all human-kind. We need not wait for total liberation, however, to attain such short-term goals as equal opportunity, maternity leave, and child care now.

APPENDIXES

APPENDIX I. A LISTING OF HEALTH HAZARDS IN SELECTED WOMEN'S OCCUPATIONS

This is an adaptation of the appendix in Stellman and Daum's *Work Is Dangerous to Your Health*. Predominantly male occupations have been eliminated, and several predominantly female occupations have been added. The reader is referred to the index for further information on many of the individual substances, and to the original book for more detailed information.

ACTRESSES AND ACTORS
  Cobalt and compounds
ADHESIVE MAKERS AND USERS
See also Glue makers and users; Gum makers; Rubber cement makers and users
  Benzene
  Chromium compounds
  Dioxane (diethylene ether)
  Ethyl silicate
  Ethylenediamine
  Fluorides
  Ketones: acetone, butanone
  Methyl alcohol
  Plastics
    Amino resins: urea-formaldehyde resins, melamine-formaldehyde resins
    Diisocyanate resins
    Epoxy resins
    Styrene
    Toluene diisocyanate (TDI)
  Pyridine
  Xylene
  Zinc compounds

AGRICULTURAL WORKERS
See Farmers and agricultural workers
AIRCRAFT-MANUFACTURE WORKERS
  Chlorinated solvents
  Chromates
  Chromic acid
  Cutting fluids
  Cyanides
  Dichromates
  Glass fibers
  Hydraulic fluids: dichromates
  Hydrogen cyanide
  Hydrogen fluoride
  Lubricants
  Nitric acid
  Oils
  Paints and thinners
  Plastics, including toluene diisocyanate (TDI)
  Radiation: ultraviolet, X-ray
  Resins, including epoxy
  Rubber antioxidants and accelerators

Solvents
Vibrating tools
Welding fumes

ANIMAL LAB WORKERS
See Hospital and laboratory
    workers: animal lab workers

AUTO-MANUFACTURE WORKERS
Abrasive dusts
Antifreeze fluids: dichromates
Brake fluids: bisphenol A, hy-
    droquinone
Carbon monoxide
Cutting fluids
Epoxy resins
Gasoline
Graphite
Lead
Lubricants
Metal cleaners, including ox-
    alic acid
Oils
Paint thinners: turpentine
Paints
Phthalic anhydride, polyester
    resins
Plastics
Rubber antioxidants and ac-
    celerators
Soldering fluxes
Solvents: chlorinated hydrocar-
    bons, methyl alcohol

BACTERIOCIDE MAKERS AND
USERS
See also Detergent makers; Soap
    makers
Fluorides
Mercury and compounds
Ozone
Silver and compounds
Tin and compounds

BAKERS
See Food processors and handlers

BARBERS AND HAIRDRESSERS
See Cosmetologists, barbers, and
    hairdressers

BATTERY MAKERS AND
WORKERS
See also Electrical and electronics
    workers; Plastic makers: resin
    makers
Amyl acetate (storage)
Antimony and compounds
    (storage)
Benzene (dry)
Cadmium (storage)
Carbolic acid
Chromium compounds (dry)
Coal tar and fractions (poly-
    cyclic hydrocarbons; dry)
Copper and compounds
Glass fibers
Graphite (dry)
Hydrogen chloride
Lead
Manganese compounds
Mercury
Nickel and compounds (stor-
    age)
Phenol (dry)
Picric acid
Plastics: epoxy resins, harden-
    ers
Silver and compounds
Sulfuric acid (storage)
Zinc chloride (dry)

BOOKBINDERS
See also Glue makers and users;
    Ink makers; Lithographers;
    Paper workers; Printers;
    Typographers, electrotypers,
    and stenotypers
Acrolein
Amyl acetate
Asbestos
Formaldehyde
Glues (plastics)
Inks (acrylic monomer, cobalt,
    methyl salicylate, resin,
    rubber, carbon black)
Lead
Methyl alcohol

Paper dust
Shellac

BUTCHERS, MEAT HANDLERS, AND SLAUGHTERHOUSE WORKERS
See also Food processors
Antibiotics
Cold
Detergents (synthetic)
Hydrogen sulfide
Infections
    Bacteria: anthrax, brucellosis, tularemia
    Fungi

CARPET MAKERS
See also Textile workers
Alizarin
Aniline dyes
Bacteria infection: anthrax
Bleach (chlorine)
Cleaners
    Formaldehyde
    para-dichlorobenzene
    Oils
Detergents
Fungicides
Glues (adhesives)
Insecticides
Loom oils
Soaps
Solvents: turpentine

CASHIERS AND TELLERS
See also Office and clerical workers
Infection
Standing: varicose veins
Ultraviolet radiation

CELLOPHANE FILM MAKERS
Acrylonitrile
Carbon disulfide
Cobalt
Dimethylamine
Ethylene glycol
Ethylene oxide
Fluorocarbons
Hydrogen sulfide

Sodium hydroxide
Sulfuric acid

CELLULOID MAKERS
Dinitrobenzene
Ethylene dibromide
Ketones
Naphthalene
Oxalic acid

CERAMIC MAKERS AND WORKERS
See also Enamel makers and workers; Pottery makers and workers
Acetylene
Aluminum and compounds
Antimony and compounds
Arsenic
Barium and compounds
Bismuth and compounds
Cadmium
Calcium oxide
Ceramic molding
Chromium and compounds
Cobalt and compounds
Fluorides
Freon
Hydroquinone
Lead
Manganese compounds
Mercury and compounds
Molybdenum and compounds
Nickel compounds
Oxalic acid
Phosphoric acid
Platinum and compounds
Selenium compounds
Silver and compounds
Tellurium compounds
Thorium and compounds
Tin and compounds
Uranium and compounds
Vanadium and compounds
X-rays
Zinc compounds

CLEANING COMPOUND MAKERS
ortho-dichlorobenzene

Ethyl alcohol
Ethylene dichloride
Ketones

CLERICAL WORKERS
See Office and clerical workers

CLINICAL LABORATORY
WORKERS
See Hospital and laboratory
workers

CLOTHING WORKERS
See Textile workers

COBBLERS AND CEMENTERS OF
RUBBER SHOES
See also Leather workers
Adhesives
Benzene
Carbon disulfide
Coal tar products
Glues
Methyl alcohol
Naphthalene
Polish

COMPOSITORS
See also Ink makers; Lithographers; Paper workers; Photoengravers; Photographic chemical makers and users; Printers
Alkalies
Aniline and derivatives
Inks
Metals
Solvents

COMPUTER OPERATORS
CRTS: eyestrain, noise

COSMETICS MAKERS
See also Perfume makers
Aluminum
Asbestos
Beeswax
Bismuth and compounds
Carnuba wax
Cellosolves
Cobalt compounds
Dioxane

Ethyl alcohol
Ethylene glycol
Fruit and vegetable oils and acids
Hexachlorophene
Isopropyl alcohol
Ketones
Lanolin
Parabens
n-propyl alcohol
Talc
Titanium compounds
Zinc compounds

COSMETOLOGISTS, BARBERS,
AND HAIRDRESSERS
Bleaches
Cosmetics
Ethanolamine
Talc
Depilatory agents: calcium thioglycolate
Dyes
Hydroquinone
Resorcinol
Styrene
p-toluenediamine
Hair lacquers
Dimethylhydantoin
Fluorocarbons
Formaldehyde resin
Polyvinyl acetate copolymer
Polyvinyl pyrrolidone
Shellac
Nail varnishes
Acetone
Acetylcellulose
Benzene
Benzyl alcohol
Ethyl alcohol
Pentyl alcohol
Plasticizers
Resins
Toluene
Xylene
Noise
Perfumes: simple or complex aromatic aldehydes
Permanent waves
Acetic acid

Alkaline sulphite
Perborates
Thioglycolate solution
Propellants
Shampoos
  Ammonium lauryl sulphite
  Triethanolamine
Ultraviolet light
Vibrating machines

DEGREASERS
See also Metal degreasers
Benzene
Carbon disulfide
Carbon tetrachloride
Dichloroethyl ethers
Diethylene tetramine
Dioxane
Methylene chloride
Perchloroethylene
Sodium and potassium hydroxides
Stripping agents: coal tar fractions
Trichloroethylene

DENTAL PRODUCTS MAKERS,
DENTAL TECHNICIANS, AND
DENTISTS
Alpha rays (uranium in dentures)
Anesthetics: ethyl chloride, nitrous oxide
Cadmium (in amalgam)
Disinfectants (aromatics)
Germanium (in alloys)
Infections, especially hepatitis
Lead (in alloys)
Mercury (in alloys)
Methylene chloride
Natural oils
  Eugenol
  Menthol
  Peppermint
  Wintergreen
Noise: high frequency (drills)
Phosphoric acid
Plastics: acrylic resins
Platinum (in alloys)

Silica (denture powder)
Soaps
X-rays
Zinc compounds (in cement)

DENTIFRICE MAKERS
Fluorides
Zinc compounds

DEODORANT MAKERS AND
USERS
See also Cosmetics makers; Drug makers
Bismuth compounds
Chloride of lime (calcium chloride, calcium hydroxide, calcium hydrochloride)
Cresol
ortho-dichlorobenzene
para-dichlorobenzene
Dioxane
Formaldehyde
Hexachlorophene
Zinc compounds
Zirconium compounds

DEPILATORY MAKERS AND
USERS
Beeswax
Hydrogen sulfide
Rosin
Thallium compounds
Thioglycolic acid

DETERGENT MAKERS
See also Soap makers
Benzene
n-butyl alcohol
Dioxane
Ethyl alcohol
Ethylene oxide
Naphtha (polycyclic hydrocarbons)
Oxalic acid
Perchloroethylene
Phosphoric acid
Silica
Sodium and potassium hydroxide
Sodium silicate

Sulfuric acid
Toluene

DIESEL ENGINE WORKERS, OPERATORS REPAIRPERSONS
Acrolein
Carbon monoxide
Chromium compounds
Coal tar and fractions (polycyclic hydrocarbons)
Sulfur dioxide

DISINFECTANT MAKERS AND USERS
See also Detergent makers
Acetaldehyde
Aniline and derivatives
Barium and compounds
Benzyl chloride (germicide)
Bismuth and compounds
Carbon dioxide
Chloride of lime (calcium chloride, calcium hydroxide, calcium hypochlorite)
Chlorine
Coal tar fractions
Cresol
Ethyl alcohol
Ethylene oxide
Fluoride compounds
Formaldehyde
Furfural (furfuraldehyde)
Hydrogen cyanide
Hydrogen peroxide
Iodine
Mercury and compounds
Methyl silicate
Nickel and compounds
Paradichlorobenzene
Phenol
Phthalic anhydride
Picric acid
Pine oil
n-propyl alcohol
Sulfur dioxide
Surfactants

Trichloroethylene
Zinc compounds

DOMESTIC WORKERS
See Service and household workers

DRUG MAKERS
Acetaldehyde
Acetonitrile
Acrolein
Allyl alcohol
Ammonia
Amyl alcohol
Aniline and derivatives
Arsenic
Barium and compounds
Benzene
Benzyl chloride
Bismuth and compounds
Bromine
n-butylamine
Carbon dioxide
Chlorinated hydrocarbons
Chromium compounds
Cobalt and compounds
Diacetone alcohol
Dimethyl formamide
Dimethyl sulfate
Ethyl acetate
Ethyl bromide
Ethyl chloride
Ethyl ether
Ethylene chlorohydrin
Ethylene dibromide
Ethylene glycol
Formaldehyde
Freons
Hexamethylenetetramine
Hydrogen bromide
Hydrogen chloride
Hydrogen peroxide
Hydroquinone
Isopropyl alcohol
Ketones
Manganese compounds
Mercury compounds

Methyl alcohol
Methyl bromide
Methyl chloride
Methylene chloride
Molybdenum compounds
Nitric acid
Nitroglycerin
Nitrophenols
Penicillin allergies
Perchloroethylene
Phenylhydrazine
Phosphoric acid
Phthalic anhydride
Picric acid
Platinum and compounds
n-propyl alcohols
Pyridine
Radiation
   Ionizing radiation
   Microwaves
   Ultraviolet radiation
Selenium
Silver and compounds
Sulfur monochloride
Sulfuric acid
Talc
Thallium and compounds
Toluene
Trichloroethylene
Turpentine
Xylene
Zirconium compounds

DRY CLEANERS
Amyl acetate
Benzene
Carbon disulfide
Carbon tetrachloride
Cellosolves
Chlorinated benzenes
Coal tar fractions (naphtha)
Dichloroethylene
Ethyl ether
Methyl alcohol
Methyl chloroform
Perchloroethylene
Propylene dichloride
Trichloroethylene

DYERS AND DYE MAKERS
Acetic acid
Acetic anhydride
Alkalies
Amines
Aniline
Antimony compounds
Benzene
Bismuth compounds
Calcium salts, calcium oxide, chloride of lime
Carbon dioxide
Cellosolves
Chlorinated benzenes
Chlorinated hydrocarbons
Chromates
Coal tar products (polycyclic hydrocarbons)
Copper and compounds
Cresol
Ethylene
Formaldehyde
Formic acid
Gums
Hydrochloric acid
Hydrogen cyanide
Hydrogen peroxide
Hydrogen sulfide
Hydroquinone
Lead compounds
Manganese compounds
Mercaptans
Molybdenum compounds
Naphthalene
beta-naphthylamine
Nickel compounds
Nitric acid
Nitrophenols
Oxalic acids
Phenylhydrazine
Phosgene
Phosphoric acid
Phthalic anhydride
Picric acid
Pyridine (textile dyeing)
Solvents
   Amyl acetate

Dimethyl formamide (DMF)
Dimethyl sulfate
Dioxane
Ethylene chlorohydrin
Ethylene glycol
Methyl alcohol
Sulfur monochloride (textile dyeing)
Sulfuric acid
Thallium compounds
Tin compounds
Vanadium
Zinc

ELECTRICAL AND ELECTRONICS WORKERS, INCLUDING APPLIANCE AND SCIENTIFIC EQUIPMENT MAKERS

See also Solder makers; Vacuum tube makers
Aluminum compounds
Asbestos
Beryllium and compounds
Bismuth compounds (for fuses)
Boron trifluoride (for nuclear instruments)
Cadmium (in solder flux)
Chlorinated biphenyls and naphthalenes (PCB's)
Coal tar and fractions
Germanium
Graphite
Ketones
Lead
Mercury and compounds
Naphthalene
Osmium and compounds
Plastics
    Allyl resins
    Diisocyanate resins (for refrigerators and freezers)
    Epoxy resins
    Fluorocarbons
    Phenolic resins
    Polyurethane (for refrigerators and freezers)
Platinum and compounds
Radiation

Infrared
Ionizing (in radar tube manufacture)
Microwaves
Ultraviolet
Selenium (in rectifiers)
Silver
Tellurium
Thallium (in infrared instruments)
Thorium
Titanium and compounds
Trichloroethylene
Welding fumes
Xylene (for quartz crystal oscillators)
Zinc

ELECTRICAL AND ELECTRONICS WORKERS: SEMI-CONDUCTOR MAKERS

See also Electrical and electronics workers
Arsenic
Bismuth and compounds
Carbon tetrachloride
Germanium and compounds
Phosphorus (white or yellow)
Selenium and compounds
Tellurium and compounds

EMBALMERS
Bacterial infections
Barium and compounds
Fluorides
Formaldehyde
Ionizing radiation
Methyl alcohol

EMULSIFYING AGENT MAKERS AND WORKERS
n-butylamine
Dioxane (diethylene ether)
Ethylenediamine
Styrene

ENAMEL MAKERS AND WORKERS

See also Pottery makers and workers

Amyl acetate
Arsenic
Barium and compounds
Benzene
Bismuth and compounds (in luminous enamel)
n-butyl acetate
Carbon disulfide
Cellosolves
Cerium (in vitreous enamel)
Chromium compounds
Cresol
Fluorides (in vitreous enamel)
Hydrogen chloride
Hydrogen fluoride (for enamel etching)
Lead
Manganese compounds
Nickel and compounds
Phthalic anhydride
Sodium and potassium hydroxide
Titanium
Toluene
Xylene
Zinc compounds
Zirconium compounds

ENGRAVERS
See also Metal workers
Cadmium
Defective illumination
Lead (in steel engraving)
Phosphoric acid
Sodium and potassium hydroxide

ETCHERS
See also Metal workers
Acids
Alkalies
Arsine
Chromium compounds
Hydrogen fluoride
Phenol
Silver compounds (for ivory etching)
Zinc compounds

EXPLOSIVES WORKERS, INCLUDING DETONATORS, CLEANERS, FILLERS AND PACKERS, SMOKELESS POWDER MAKERS
Acetaldehyde
Acetic anhydride
Ammonia and salts
Amyl acetate (in smokeless powder)
Amyl alcohol
Aniline and derivatives
Barium compounds
Benzene
Carbon dioxide
Carbon disulfide
Cerium
Chromium compounds
Cresol
Dinitrobenzene
Dinitrophenol
Dinitrotoluene
Ethyl acetate (in smokeless powder)
Ethyl alcohol
Ethyl ether
Ethylene glycol
Graphite
Hexamethylenetetramine
Hydrazine
Ketones
Mercury and compounds
Methyl alcohol
Naphthalene (in smokeless powder)
Nitric acid
Nitrobenzene
Nitroglycerine
Nitrophenols
PETN
Phenol
Picric acid
Pyridine
Sulfuric acid
Tetryl
Toluene
Trinitrotoluene (TNT)
Zirconium

FARMERS AND AGRICULTURAL
WORKERS
See also Fertilizer makers and
    users; Pesticide and insecti-
    cide makers and users
    Ammonia (corn growing)
    Arsenic
    Asbestos
    Bacterial infections
    Calcium cyanamide (in fertil-
        izer
    Calcium oxide
    Coal tar and fractions (poly-
        cyclic hydrocarbons)
    Cold
    Detergents (synthetic)
    Ethylene dibromide (cabbage
        growers)
    Feeds
    Fertilizers
    Fluorides (vegetable growers)
    Fruits (allergies)
    Fungus infections
    Heat
    Kerosene
    Lead
    Lubricants
    Mercury compounds
    Oils
    Parasitic infections
    Pesticides
    Poisonous plants
    Ragweed
    Solvents
    Sunlight
    Vegetables (allergies)
    Virus and rickettsial infections
FARMING AND AGRICULTURAL
WORK: SEED HANDLERS AND
PROCESSORS
    Carbon tetrachloride (in ex-
        traction of seed oils)
    Ethylene dibromide (as insec-
        ticide)
    Hexachlorobenzene (as seed
        disinfectant)

Mercury compounds (as insec-
    ticide)
Selenium and compounds (for
    germination testing)
Tetramethylthiuram disulfide
    (as disinfectant)
Zinc compounds (in seed treat-
    ment)
FARMING AND AGRICULTURAL
WORK: SOIL TREATMENT
    Carbon disulfide
    Chlorobenzenes
    Ethylene dibromide (as fumi-
        gant)
    Fluorides
    Methyl bromide (as fumigant)
    Naphthalene
    Tetrachloroethane
FEATHER WORKERS
    Aniline and derivatives
    Hydrogen peroxide
    Methyl alcohol
FEED MAKERS (ANIMAL FEEDS)
    Cobalt compounds (in mineral
        feeds)
    Manganese compounds
    Phosphoric acid
    Zinc compounds (as additives)
FELT MAKERS AND WORKERS
    Acids
    Coal tar and fractions (poly-
        cyclic hydrocarbons)
    Dyes
    Hydrogen peroxide
    Hydrogen sulfide
    Mercuric nitrate
    Methyl alcohol
    Sodium carbonate
FERTILIZER MAKERS AND
USERS: AGRICULTURAL
CHEMICALS
    Ammonia and compounds
    Arsine
    Bacterial infections: anthrax
    Calcium cyanamide
    Calcium oxide

Cobalt and compounds (in hydrogenation of oils)
Cycloparaffins
Dichloroethyl ether
1,2-dichloroethylene
Ethyl chloride
Ethyl ether
Ethylene dibromide
Ethylene dichloride
Hydrogen peroxide
Hydrogen sulfide
Hydroquinone
Infections: bacteria (anthrax)
Isopropyl acetate
Methylene chloride
Natural gas (in hydrogenation of oils)
Nickel (in hydrogenation of oils)
Nitroparaffins
Ozone (in bleaching)
Petroleum naphtha
Propylene dichloride
Sodium and potassium hydroxide (in vegetable oil processing)
Tetrachloroethane
Trichloroethylene

FOOD PROCESSORS: MEAT PACKERS
See Butchers, meat handlers, and slaughterhouse workers

FOOD PROCESSORS: SACCHARIN MAKERS
Phosphorus trichloride
Saccharin
Toluene

FOOD PROCESSORS: SUGAR PROCESSING AND REFINING
Ammonia
Bagasse (sugar cane)
Calcium oxide
Carbon dioxide
Chlorine
Hydrogen chloride
Hydrogen sulfide (in sugar-beet processing)
Methyl alcohol
Phosphoric acid
Sulfur dioxide
Sulfuric acid
Sulfur monochloride
Tin and compounds

FOOD PROCESSORS: VEGETABLE OIL EXTRACTION AND PURIFICATION
Acetonitrile
Barium and compounds
Chlorinated biphenyls and naphthalenes (PCB's)
Methyl bromide
n-propyl alcohol
Sodium and potassium hydroxide
Sulfur monochloride

FOOD PROCESSORS: YEAST MAKERS
Acetaldehyde
Carbon dioxide
Hydrogen fluoride
Phosphoric acid

FURNITURE WORKERS
Amyl acetate (in polish)
Benzene
Chromium compounds
Dichloroethyl ether (in finish remover)
Formaldehyde
Lacquers
Methyl alcohol
Microwave radiation (in veneering)
Petroleum fractions: benzene, naphtha
Plastics: amino resins, toluene diisocyanate (TDI)
Pyridine
Rosin
Soaps
Sodium and potassium hydroxide

Turpentine
Waxes
Woods
FURNITURE WORKERS:
UPHOLSTERERS
Adhesives
Bacterial infections: anthrax
Glues
Lacquer solvents
Methyl alcohol
Stains
Toluene diisocyanate (TDI)
Varnish
GLUE MAKERS AND USERS
See also Adhesive makers and
users; Gum makers; Rubber
cement makers and users
Ammonia
Bacterial infections: anthrax,
folliculitis
Benzene
Carbon dioxide
Carbon disulfide
Chromium compounds
Copper and compounds
Cresols
Dioxane (diethylene ether)
Ethylene glycol
GUM MAKERS
Cellosolves
Chlorinated biphenyls and
napththalenes (PCB's)
ortho-dichlorobenzene
Dichloroethyl ether
1,2-dichloroethylene
Epichlorohydrin
Ethyl ether
Isopropyl alcohol
Perchloroethylene
Propylene dichloride
Toluene
HERBICIDE MAKERS AND USERS
Allyl alcohol
Ammonium sulfamate (am-
mate)
Arsenic

Asbestos
Benzene
Calcium cyanamide
2,4,-D (2,4-dichlorophenoxyace-
tic acid)
Dinitrophenol
Pentachlorophenol
Phenol
Phenylmercuric acetate
Phthalic anhydride
2,4,5-T (2,4,5-trichlorophenoxy-
acetic acid)
HOSPITAL AND LABORATORY
WORKERS, INCLUDING AIDES,
DOCTORS, AND NURSES
Anesthetics
Ethyl bromide
Ethyl chloride
Ethyl ether
Halothane
Methoxyfluorane
Nitrous oxide
Antibiotics
Antiseptics
Beryllium
Cobalt
Detergents (synthetic)
Disinfectants and germicides
Drugs
Fumigants
Infections
Bacteria
Viruses, especially hepatitis
Iodine
Isopropyl alcohol
Lacerations
Lifting: back injuries
Moisture
Puncture wounds
Radiation
Gamma rays
Ionizing
Ultraviolet radiation
X-rays
Soaps
Talc
Tricresyl phosphate (in steri-
lizing surgical instruments)

Copper and compounds
Cresols
Diacetone alcohol (in quick-drying inks)
Ethyl acetate
Ethyl alcohol
Ethylene glycol
Formaldehyde
Isopropyl alcohol
Ketones
Manganese compounds
Mercury and compounds
Methyl alcohol
Nickel and compounds
Oxalic acid
Platinum and compounds (in indelible inks)
Selenium and compounds
Silver and compounds (in indelible inks)
Toluene
Turpentine
Vanadium
Xylene
Zinc compounds

INK REMOVER MAKERS AND USERS
See also Ink makers
Cresols
Oxalic acid

INSECTICIDE MAKERS AND USERS
See Farmers and agricultural workers; Pesticide and insecticide makers and users

JEWELRY MAKERS AND WORKERS, JEWELERS
Amyl acetate
Arsine
Chromium compounds
Hydrogen chloride
Hydrogen cyanide
Lead
Mercury and compounds
Nitric acid
Platinum

Silver
Sulfuric acid

KEYPUNCH OPERATORS
Dust
Noise
Wrist strain (tenosynovitis)

LABORATORY WORKERS
See Hospital and laboratory workers

LACQUER MAKERS AND USERS
Acetaldehyde
Ammonia
Amyl acetate
Amyl alcohol
Benzene
n-butyl acetate
n-butyl alcohol
Carbon disulfide
Carbon tetrachloride
Cellosolves
Chlorinated benzenes
Chlorinated biphenyls and naphthalenes (PCB's)
Cobalt and compounds
Cycloparaffins
Diacetone alcohol
Dichloroethyl ether
Dioxane (diethylene ether)
Epichlorohydrin
Ethyl acetate
Ethyl benzene
Ethyl ether
Ethylene chlorohydrin
Ethylene dichloride
Ethylene glycol
Formaldehyde
Infrared radiation
Isopropyl alcohol
Ketones
Methyl alcohol
Methylene chloride
Nitric acid
Plastics: alkyd resins, phenolic resins
Propyl acetate
n-propyl alcohol

Pyridine
Tetrachloroethane
Titanium and compounds
Toluene
Trichloroethylene
Turpentine
Xylene
Zirconium compounds

LAUNDRY WORKERS
Acetic acid
Bacteriocides
Bleaches: chloride of lime, chlorine
Detergents (synthetic)
Dusts and toxic contaminants
Fluorides
Formic acid
Heat
Hydrogen fluorides
Infections
Lacerations
Mechanical injuries
Oxalic acid
Soaps
Sodium and potassium hydroxides

LEATHER WORKERS
Acrylonitrile (in finishing)
Amyl acetate
Aniline and derivatives
Antimony and compounds: mordanters
Arsenic
Benzene
n-butyl acetate (in glue or dope)
Cellosolves (ethylene glycol derivatives)
Chromium compounds (in tanning)
Ethyl acetate
Ethylene glycol dyers
Formic acid
Methylene chloride (in finishes)

Oxalic acid (as bleach)
Xylene

LEATHER WORKERS (ARTIFICIAL LEATHER)
Isopropyl acetate
Ketones
Monomers
Plastics (vinyls)
Polyvinyl acetate
Polyvinyl alcohol
Polyvinyl chloride

LIBRARIANS
Dust
Asbestos
Spores (allergies)
Talc

LITHOGRAPHERS
See also Ink makers; Paper workers; Photoengravers; Printers
Aluminum and compounds
Aniline and derivatives
Benzene
Cadmium
Chromium compounds
Copper and compounds
Formaldehyde
Hydrogen chloride
Hydrogen sulfide
Hydroquinone
Inks
Lead
Mercuric chlorine
Methyl alcohol
Nitric acid
Oxalic acid
Phosphoric acid
Photographic fluids
Sodium and potassium hydroxide
Talc
Turpentine
Ultraviolet radiation
Xylene

MATCH MAKERS
Ammonium phosphate
Antimony and compounds
Barium and compounds

Carbon disulfide
Chromates
Dextrins
Dyes
Formaldehyde
Glues
Graphite
Gums
Lead
Manganese
Phosphorus pentachloride
Phosphorus sesquisulfide
Picric acid
Potassium chlorate
Sodium and potassium hydroxide
Thallium and compounds
Zinc compounds

MEAT WORKERS
See Butchers, meat handlers, and slaughterhouse workers

MEAT WRAPPERS
See also Butchers, meat handlers, and slaughterhouse workers
Cold and dampness
Decomposition of meat wrap
Carbon monoxide
Chlorine
Hydrochloric acid
Phosgene

METAL CLEANERS, POLISHERS, BURNISHERS, COATERS, AND CONDITIONERS; MAKERS AND USERS OF POLISHING SUBSTANCES
See also Metal degreasers; Polish makers and users
Abrasive dusts: silica, silicates, corundum, etc.
Ammonia
Arsine
Chromium compounds
Detergents
Diethylenetriamine
Fluorides
Freons

Hydrogen chloride
Hydrogen cyanide
Hydrogen fluoride
Hydrogen peroxide
Kerosene
Metal dusts
Nitrogen dioxide
Oxalic acid
Petroleum naphtha
Phosphoric acid
Solvents (for degreasing)
Carbon tetrachloride
Diacetone alcohol
Dichlorobenzene
Dioxane (diethylene ether)
Ethylene glycol
Ketones
Methyl alcohol
Nitrobenzene
Sulfuric acid
Trichloroethane
Trichloroethylene
Triethanolamine
Waxes
Zinc compounds (in steel polish)

METAL DEGREASERS
Chlorinated benzenes
Chlorinated biphenyls and naphthalenes (PCB's)
Ethylene dichloride
Methyl chloroform
Naphtha (petroleum distillate)
Perchloroethylene
Propyl acetate
n-propyl alcohol
Trichloroethane
Trichloroethylene

METAL ETCHERS
See Etchers

METAL PLATERS, ELECTROPLATERS
See also Metal workers
Ammonia
Antimony and compounds (as metal bronzers)
Arsine

Barium and compounds
Bismuth and compounds
Cadmium
Calcium
Calcium oxide
Carbon disulfide
Chlorinated biphenyls and
    naphthalenes (PCB's)
Chromic acid, chromium com-
    pounds
Cobalt and compounds
Copper and compounds
Detergents
Fluorides
Formic acid
Graphite
Hydrogen chloride
Hydrogen cyanide
Hydrogen peroxide
Lead
Mercury and compounds
Nickel carbonyl (gas platers)
Nickel compounds
Nitrogen dioxide
Platinum and compounds
Selenium and compounds
Soaps
Sodium and potassium hydrox-
    ides
Titanium
Waxes (synthetic)
Zinc and compounds

**METAL WORKERS: RUST RE-
MOVERS, RUST PROOFERS**
Abrasives: silica, corundum
Chromates
Decaborane (as rust inhibitor)
Oxalic acid (as rust remover)
Phosphoric acid (as rust inhibi-
    tor)
Pyridine (as rust inhibitor)
Tetrachloroethane (as rust re-
    mover)

MILLINERY WORKERS
Aniline and derivatives

Benzene
Methyl alcohol

MORDANTERS
See also Dyers and dye makers
Acids
Alkalies
Aluminum salts
Amyl alcohol
Antimony compounds
Arsenates
Barium (in textile dyeing)
Chromium salts
Copper salts
Fluorides (in textile dyeing)
Formaldehyde

**NAIL ENAMEL AND POLISH
MAKERS**
See Cosmetics makers

**NUCLEAR REACTOR WORKERS
AND NUCLEAR TECHNOLOGISTS**
Beryllium and compounds
Cobalt and compounds
Graphite
Ionizing radiation
Lead
Thorium and compounds
Uranium and compounds
Zirconium compounds

NYLON MAKERS
See Textile workers: nylon makers

**OFFICE AND CLERICAL
WORKERS**
Adhesives
Air-conditioned air impurities
    Asbestos
    Fibrous glass
    Fungal spores (causing allergy)
Duplicating-fluid removers
Duplicating materials
Ink removers
Inks
Noise
Ozone
Rubber
Solvents

Ammonia
Amyl acetate (for coated paper)
Arsine
Asbestos
Bagasse (sugar cane)
Barium and compounds
n-butyl acetate (for coated paper)
Calcium oxide
Chloride of lime
Chlorinated biphenyls and naphthalenes (for treated paper, carbonless carbon paper)
Chlorine
Chromium compounds (for paper dyeing)
Diacetone alcohol
Formaldehyde
Formic acid
Graphite
Hydrogen sulfide (pulp workers)
Oxalic acid
Plastics: amino resins for paper treaters
Selenium compounds
Sodium and potassium hydroxide
Sulfur dioxide
Sulfuric acid
Tin and compounds (in sensitized paper)
Titanium
Trichloroethylene (in paper cups)
Zinc compounds

PENCIL MAKERS
Adhesives and glues
Aniline and derivatives (colored pencils)
Benzene
Chromates (in colored pencils)
Graphite
Lacquer thinners

Methyl violet
Pyridine
Red cedar wood
Resins
Solvents
Waxes

PERFUME MAKERS
See also Cosmetics makers
Acetaldehyde
Acetic anhydride
Acetonitrile
Acrolein (acrylic aldehyde)
Ammonia
Amyl acetate
Amyl alcohol
Aniline and derivatives
Benzene
Benzyl chloride
Bismuth and compounds
n-butyl acetate
Cellosolves
Chlorinated benzenes
Chromium compounds
Cresol
Cycloparaffins
1,2-dichloroethylene
Dimethyl sulfate
Ethyl acetate
Ethyl chloride
Ethyl ether
Formic acid
Isopropyl acetate
Methyl alcohol
Methylene chloride
Phenol
Propyl acetate
Sodium and potassium hydroxide
Tin and compounds
Toluene
Trichloroethylene

PESTICIDE AND INSECTICIDE MAKERS AND USERS
Acetic acid
Arsenic
Asbestos

Barium and compounds
Benzene
n-butylamine
Calcium oxide
Carbon dioxide
Carbon tetrachloride
Cellosolves
Chlorinated benzenes
    ortho-dichlorobenzene
    para-dichlorobenzene
    Trichlorobenzene
Chlorinated diphenyls and
    naphthalenes
Coal tar and fractions (poly-
    cyclic hydrocarbons)
Copper and compounds
Cresols
Ethylene chlorohydrin
Ethylene dibromide
Ethylene dichloride
Ethylene oxide
Fluorides
Formic acid
Hydrazine
Hydrogen cyanide
Kerosene
Lead
Mercury
Methyl bromide
Methyl formate
Naphtha (petroleum distillate)
Naphthalene
Phosphorus (white and yellow)
Phosphorus pentasulfide
Phthalic anhydride
Sulfur monochloride
Tetrachloroethane
Tetramethylthiuram disulfide
Thallium and compounds
Toluene
Xylene
Zinc compounds

PHOTOENGRAVERS

See also Ink makers; Lithogra-
    phers; Paper workers; Pho-
    tographic chemical makers
    and users; Printers

Ammonia
Amyl acetate
Chromates
High-intensity light
Hydrogen cyanide
Hydrogen sulfide
Methyl alcohol
Nitric acid
Oxalic acid
Ozone
Phosphoric acid
Sodium and potassium hydrox-
    ide
Ultraviolet radiation

PHOTOGRAPHIC CHEMICAL MAKERS AND USERS

Acetaldehyde
Acetic acid
Ammonia (automatic film
    processing)
Amyl alcohol
Aniline and derivatives
Barium and compounds
Benzene
Benzyl chloride (in developers)
Bromine
Chlorine (in developers)
Chromates
Cresol (in developers)
Dimethyl hydrazine (in devel-
    opers)
Dinitrophenol (in developers)
Hydrogen peroxide (in devel-
    opers)
Hydroquinone (in developers)
Light: high intensity, photo-
    graphing
Mercury compounds
Nitrophenols
Oxalic acid
Ozone (photographers)
Petroleum naphtha
Phenol
Quinone (in developers)
Selenium
Silver compounds

Sulfuric acid
Trichloroethylene (plate cleaners)
Trinitrotoluene (TNT)
Uranium and compounds
Vanadium

PIGMENT MAKERS AND USERS
Antimony and compounds
Arsenic
Barium and compounds
Bismuth and compounds
Cadmium and compounds
Chromates
Copper and compounds
Graphite
Hydrogen chloride
Hydrogen cyanide

PLASTIC MAKERS: RESIN MAKERS
See also Plastic makers; Plasticizer makers and users
Acetaldehyde
Acrolein (acrylic aldehyde)
Allyl alcohol
Ammonia
Benzene
Benzyl chloride
Carbon disulfide
Cellosolves
Chlorinated benzenes
Chlorinated biphenyls and naphthalenes (PCB's)
Cresol
Cycloparaffins
Decaborane
Diacetone alcohol
Dichloroethyl ether
1,2,-dichloroethylene
Dimethyl formamide
Dioxane (diethylene ether)
Ethyl acetate
Ethyl benzene
Ethyl chloride
Ethylene chloride
Ethylene chlorohydrin

Ethylene dichloride
Ethylene glycol
Formaldehyde
Furfural (furfuraldehyde)
Hexamethylenetetramine
Isopropyl acetate
Ketones
Methyl alcohol
Methylene chloride
Mineral oil
Naphthalene
Nitroparaffins
Oils: cashew nut oil, mineral oil
Phenol
Phosgene
Phthalic anhydride
Plastic resins
    Alkyd resins
    Allyl resins
    Amino resins
    Diisocyanate resins
    Epoxy resins
    Phenolic resins
    Polyester resins
Propyl acetate
n-propyl alcohol
Tetrachloroethane
Titanium and compounds
Toluene
Trichloroethylene
Turpentine
Xylene

PLASTIC MAKERS
Acetaldehyde (in phenolic resins)
Acetic acids
Acetic anhydride
Acetone
Acetonitrile; plasticizers and polymethylacrylic resins
Acrylic resins
Alkyd resins
Allyl alcohol
Allyl resins
Aluminum compounds
Amino resins

Ammonia
Amyl acetate
Amyl alcohol
Aniline and derivatives
Arsine
Asbestos
n-butyl alcohol (in plasticizers)
Cellulosics
Chlorinated diphenyls and
    naphthalenes
Cobalt and compounds (in
    polyester resins)
Cresol
Cycloparaffins (for molding
    plastic)
Diatomite
1,2-dichloroethylene
Diisocyanate resins
Dinitrobenzene
Dioxane (diethylene ether)
Epichlorohydrin
Epoxy resins
Ethyl acetate
Ethyl ether
Ethyl silicate (for protective
    coatings)
Ethylene dichloride
Ethylene oxide
Fibrous glass
Formaldehyde
Formic acid
Freon
Furfural (furfuraldehyde)
Glass fibers
Hexylmethylenetetramine
Hydrogen chloride
Hydrogen cyanide
Hydrogen fluoride
Hydrogen peroxide (in plastic
    foam)
Hydroquinone
Isopropyl acetate
Ketones
Lead
Methyl chloride (in polysty-
    rene foam)

Mica
Nylon
Organic tin compounds
Phenol
Phosgene
Phthalic anhydride
Polyester resins
Polyethylenes
Polystyrenes
Quartz
Selenium and compounds
Silica
Styrene
Tin compounds
Toluene diisocyanate (TDI)
Tricresyl phosphate (in plasti-
    cizers, polyvinyl chloride,
    polystyrene)
Vinyl chloride
Vinyl plastics
Xylene (in polyester teraph-
    thalate film)

PLASTICIZER MAKERS AND
USERS

Acrylonitrile
Allyl alcohol
n-butyl alcohol
Chlorinated biphenyls and
    naphthalenes (PCB's)
Ethylene dichloride (in plasti-
    cizer bath)
Phosphorus oxychloride
Phosphorus trichloride
Phthalic anhydride
Tricresyl phosphate

POLISH MAKERS AND WORKERS
See also Metal cleaners, polishers
Amyl acetate
Aniline and derivatives
ortho-dichlorobenzene
Dioxane (diethylene ether)
Graphite
Hydrogen cyanide
Hydrogen fluoride
Methyl alcohol
Nitrobenzene (in shoe polish)

Phosphoric acid
n-propyl alcohol
Titanium and compounds (in white shoe polish)
Trichloroethylene
Turpentine (in store enamel polishes)
Zirconium compounds

POSTAL WORKERS
Carbon monoxide
Cold
Dust
Improper illumination
Infections
Bacteria: dermatitis
Fungi: dermatitis
Lifting: back injuries
Noise

POTTERY MAKERS AND WORKERS
See also Ceramic makers and workers; Enamel makers and workers
Aluminum and compounds
Carbon dioxide
Hydrogen chloride
Lead
Talc
Zirconium compounds

PRACTICAL NURSES
See Hospital and laboratory workers

PRINTERS
See also Adhesive makers and users; Glue makers and users; Ink makers; Ink remover makers and users; Lithographers; Paper workers; Photoengravers; Photographic chemical makers and users; Textile printers; Typographers, electrotypers, and stenotypers
Aniline and derivatives

Asbestos
Benzene
Carbon black
Carbon tetrachloride
Cellosolves
Chlorinated biphenyls and naphthalenes (PCB's)
Chromates
Cornstarch
Diacetone alcohol
Dioxane (diethylene ether)
Formaldehyde
Gums: acacia, arabic
Hexane (tulosol)
Hydrogen cyanide (in textile and art printing)
Ink mists
Isopropyl alcohol
Ketones
Lead (in wallpaper printing)
Methyl alcohol
Methyl chloride
Paper dust
Sodium and potassium hydroxide
Talc
Toluene
Trichloroethylene
Urea-formaldehyde resins

PROPELLENT AND AEROSOL MAKERS AND WORKERS
Amino resins: urea-formaldehyde and melamine-formaldehyde resins
Carbon dioxide
Carbon tetrachloride
Chlorine
Freon
Methyl chloride
Methylene chloride

RESIN MAKERS
See Plastic makers: Resin makers

RETAIL SALES WORKERS
Dust
Infection

Lifting: back injuries
Noise
Standing: varicose veins
RUBBER: LATEX WORKERS
See also Rubber makers and
    workers
  Ammonia
  Fluorides
  Phosphoric acid
  Pyridine
RUBBER CEMENT MAKERS AND
USERS
  Adhesives
  Airplane dope
  Ammonia
  Amyl acetate
  Benzene
  n-butyl alcohol
  Carbon disulfide
  Gum
  Ketones
  Sulfur monochloride
  Toluene
  Trichloroethylene
  Xylene
RUBBER MAKERS AND WORKERS
  Acetaldehyde
  Acetic acid
  Acetylene
  Acrolein (acrylic aldehyde)
  Acrylonitrile
  Alkalies
  Aluminum and compounds
  Ammonia
  Amyl acetate
  Amyl alcohol
  Aniline and derivatives
  Antimony and compounds
  Benzene
  Benzidine
  Benzyl chloride
  Butadiene
  n-butylamine
  Calcium oxide
  Carbon black

Carbon disulfide
Carbon tetrachloride
Chlorinated benzenes
Chlorinated biphenyls and
    naphthalenes (PCB's)
Chlorine
Chloroprene (chlorobutadine;
    in neoprene)
Chromates
Coal tar and fractions
Cobalt and compounds (as col-
    oring)
Copper and compounds
Cresol
Cycloparaffins
Decaborane
para-dichlorobenzene
1,2-dichloroethylene
Ethyl alcohol
Ethylenediamine
Formaldehyde
Formic acid
Freon (in sponge rubber)
Furfural (furfuraldehyde)
Graphite
Hexamethylenetetramine
Hydrochloric acid
Hydroquinone (in rubber coat-
    ing)
Ketones
Lead
Manganese compounds
Mercaptans
Methyl alcohol
Methyl chloride
Methylene chloride
Oxalic acid
Perchloroethylene
Petroleum naphtha
Phenol (in reclaiming rubber)
Phosphoric acid (in rubber la-
    tex)
Phosphorus pentasulfide
Propylene dichloride
Pyridine
Selenium

Styrene
Sulfuric acid
Talc
Tellurium
Tetrachloroethane
Tetramethylthiuram disulfide
    (in heat-resistant rubber)
Titanium
Tolylene diisocyanate (in abrasion-resistant rubber)
Turpentine
Vinyl chloride
Xylene
Zinc compounds

RUBBER VULCANIZERS
Ammonia
Aniline and derivatives
Barium and compounds
Carbon dioxide
Hydrogen sulfide
Methyl alcohol
Sulfur monochloride
Tellurium
Tetramethylthiuram disulfide

SALESWOMEN
See Retail sales workers

SCIENTIFIC WORKERS AND TECHNICIANS
See Hospital and laboratory workers

SERVICE AND HOUSEHOLD WORKERS
See also Food processors; Laundry workers
Alkalies
Bending and lifting: back injuries
Detergents
Disinfectants
Infection
Kneeling: knee injuries
Noise
Standing: varicose veins
Wet hands: skin irritation

SHOEMAKERS
See also Cobblers and cementers of rubber shoes; Glue makers and users; Leather workers; Pigment makers and users; Polish makers and workers
Adhesives
Ammonia (in finishing)
Amyl acetate
Amyl alcohol
Dioxane (diethylene ether; in shoe creams)
Furfural (furfuraldehyde; in shoe dyes)
Glues
Ketones
Lead (in stains)
Methyl alcohol
Titanium and compounds (in shoe-whitening compounds)
Trichloroethylene

SOAP MAKERS
See also Bacteriocide makers and users; Detergent makers
Acrolein (acrylic aldehyde)
Alkalies
Amyl acetate
Barium and compounds
Calcium oxide
Cellosolves
Chloride of lime (as bleach)
Chromates
Cobalt compounds
Dichloroethyl ether
Ethylene dichloride
Hydrochloric acid
Hydrogen peroxide (as bleach)
Hydrogen sulfide
Methyl alcohol
Nitrobenzene

SOLDER MAKERS; SOLDER FLUX MAKERS AND USERS
Acids

Ethylendiamine (in textile lubricants)
Ethylene dichloride (in textile cleaners)
Ethylene glycol
Ethylene oxide (as fumigant and textile lubricant)
Formaldehyde (in waterproofing)
Formic acid
Hexamethylenetetramine
Hydrogen peroxide (as bleach)
Hydroquinone (as textile coating)
Ketones
Lead
Manganese compounds (as textile fiber bleach)
Nitroparaffins
Ozone (as bleach)
Plastics: alkyd resins, amino resins
Selenium
Sodium and potassium hydroxide (as bleaches)
Sulfur dioxide (as bleach)
Sulfuric acid
Thallium compounds
Tin and compounds
Toluene
Trichloroethylene (in textile cleaners)
Zinc compounds
Zirconium compounds

TEXTILE WORKERS: COTTON, THREAD, AND CLOTH WORKERS (MILLING, BLEACHING, PREPARING, AND SIZING CLOTH)

Cobalt (in making ethyl acrylate)
Copper and compounds
Diacetone alcohol
Dichloroethyl ether (in making ethyl cellulose)
1,2-dichloroethylene

Dioxane
Ethyl chloride (in making ethyl cellulose)
Ethylene chlorohydrin (in making ethyl cellulose)
Furfural (furfuraldehyde)
Hydrogen cyanide
Ketones
Methyl alcohol
Methylene chloride
Methyl formate
Nitric acid
Nitroparaffin
Perchloroethylene (in cellulose ester)
Phosphorus pentachloride (in making acetyl cellulose)
Phthalic anhydride (as plasticizer)
Sulfuric acid
Tetrachloroethane
Zinc chloride

TEXTILE WORKERS: NITROCELLULOSE MAKERS AND WORKERS

Amyl acetate
Amyl alcohol
Arsine
Benzene
n-butyl alcohol
Cellosolves
Diacetone alcohol
Ethyl acetate
Furfural (furfuraldehyde)
Isopropyl acetate
Nitroparaffins: nitroethane, nitromethane, nitropropane
Propyl acetate
n-propyl alcohol
Tricresyl phosphate

TEXTILE WORKERS: NYLON MAKERS

Cycloparaffins
Furfural (furfuraldehyde)
Hydrogen cyanide
Polyamides

TEXTILE WORKERS: RAYON
VISCOSE MAKERS

See also Cellophane film makers
  Acetonitrile
  Ammonia
  Arsine
  Asbestos
  Carbon dioxide
  Carbon disulfide
  Chlorinated biphenyls and
      naphthalenes (PCB's)
  Chlorine
  Copper and compounds
  Dimethyl amine
  Ethylene oxide
  Fluorides
  Hydrogen cyanide
  Hydrogen sulfide
  Lead (in lead burning)
  Oxalic acid (as bleach)
  Plastics: fluorocarbons
  Sodium and potassium hydrox-
      ide
  Sulfuric acid
  Zinc compounds

TEXTILE WORKERS: SILK
PROCESSERS

  Acids
  Alkalies
  Amyl acetate
  Bromine (as bleach)
  Chromates (in silk-screen mak-
      ing)
  Hydrogen peroxide (as bleach)
  Hydrogen sulfide
  Isopropyl acetate
  Nitrogen dioxide (in raw-silk
      bleaching)
  Xylene (in silk finishing)
  Zinc compounds

TEXTILE WORKERS: WOOL
PROCESSERS

  Ammonia (scourers)
  Bromine (in shrinkproofing)
  Cresol (scourers)

ortho-dichlorobenzene (in de-
    greasing)
Ethylene dibromide (reclaim-
    ers)
Ethylene dichloride (as
    cleaner)
Hydrogen peroxide (wool
    printers)
Infections
    Bacteria: anthrax, rickettsia,
    fever
    Fungi: ringworm
Methyl bromide
Perchloroethylene (scourers)
Petroleum naphtha
Sulfur dioxide (as bleach)
Trichloroethylene (scourers)

TYPOGRAPHERS, ELECTROTYP-
ERS, AND STENOTYPERS (PRINT-
ING TRADES)

See also Engravers; Ink makers;
    Lithographers; Paper work-
    ers; Printers
  Ammonia
  Antimony
  Arsenic
  Graphite
  Inks
  Lead
  Silver
  Tin
  Type-cleaning solvents

VACUUM TUBE MAKERS

See also Electrical and electronics
    workers
  Carbon disulfide
  Germanium
  Ionizing radiation
  Methyl alcohol
  Molybdenum and compounds
  Perchloroethylene
  Thorium
  Titanium
  Trichloroethylene
  Zirconium

VARNISH MAKERS AND USERS
  Acetaldehyde
  Acids
  Alkalies
  Amyl acetate
  Amyl alcohol
  Aniline and derivatives
  Barium and compounds
  n-butyl alcohol
  Carbon disulfide
  Cellosolves
  Chlorinated benzenes
  Chlorinated biphenyls and
      naphthalenes (PCB's)
  Cobalt and compounds
  Dichloroethyl ether
  Ethyl acetate
  Ethyl alcohol
  Ethylene chlorohydrin
  Ethylene dichloride
  Furfural (furfuraldehyde)
  Hydroquinone
  Isopropyl alcohol

VARNISH REMOVER MAKERS
AND USERS
See also Varnish makers and
      users
  Carbon disulfide
  Carbon tetrachloride
  Cellosolves
  Chlorinated benzenes
  Cresols
  Epichlorohydrin
  Ethylene dichloride
  Ketones
  Methylene chloride
  Oxalic acid
  Styrene
WAITRESSES
  Carrying and lifting: back in-
      juries
  Cigarette smoke
  Infection
  Noise
  Standing: varicose veins
  Wet hands: skin irritation

APPENDIX II. A QUICK GUIDE TO OBSERVED EFFECTS OF SELECTED OCCUPATIONAL HEALTH HAZARDS

A. SOLVENTS

1. *Aromatic Hydrocarbons*

Benzene

Depresses bone marrow activity which can lead to anemia and/or a deficiency in white blood cells and platelets. Also can cause leukemia. Probably has adverse effects on male and female reproductivity.

Toluene

A powerful narcotic that can seriously impair a worker's reflexes and judgment, possibly leading to an increased accident rate. Commercial toluene often is contaminated with significant levels of benzene.

Xylene

Thought to be less toxic than benzene, but not well studied. Menstrual disturbances have been reported as have various alterations of the blood cells. Should be treated with caution.

2. *Chlorinated Hydrocarbons*

Vary in toxicity from relatively harmless to potentially fatal. Anesthetic effects and adverse liver effects often noted. One should not depend on odor as a warning because the nose may become accustomed to the smell, and in many cases the odor level is higher than the legal exposure limits.

Carbon tetrachloride*

At high levels can lead to depression of nervous system functions.

	Lower levels can be seriously toxic to liver and kidneys. Serious damage and even death have followed single high-level exposures.
Methylene chloride	An extremely volatile solvent that is irritating to the eyes, nose, and throat. Acts as a narcotic and is converted by the body to carbon monoxide.
Trichloroethylene* (TCE)	Markedly affects the nervous system, leading to giddiness, dizziness, fatigue, headaches, etc. Alcoholic beverages often not tolerated. Decomposes to hydrochloric acid and phosgene when heated.
Tetrachloroethane	Extremely toxic, especially to the liver. Easily absorbed through the skin.
Tetrachloroethylene (perchloroethylene)	Narcotic effects. Liver damage reported in exposed test animals and in some studies on workers.
3. *Ketones*	At low levels members of this chemical family are mildly narcotic and irritating to the eyes, nose, and throat. MEK, methylethyl ketone, is thought to have been associated with severe nervous system defects in one factory. The irritating odor should not be ignored.
	Threshold limit value† (TLV) in parts per million (ppm)
Acetone	1000 (may not be low enough to prevent discomfort)
Methylethyl ketone (MEK)	200
Methyl isobutyl ketone (MIBK)	100 (may not be low enough to prevent discomfort)
Methyl-n-propyl ketone	200
4. *Carbon disulfide*	Used in the manufacture of viscose rayon, this is a highly irritating and

toxic substance. It can be rapidly fatal, but at lower-than-fatal levels it can damage the brain and nervous system, even leading to blindness, hallucinations, and other manifestations of mental illness. At still lower levels, workers seem to develop more heart attacks and high blood pressure at earlier ages.

B. Cancer-causing Substances in the Workplace

The National Institute for Occupational Safety and Health (NIOSH) has indentified 1,500 potentially cancer-causing substances (carcinogens) in the workplace. Following are some that may be of particular relevance to women.

Substance	Cancer Site	Some Potential Occurrences
Asbestos	Lung, chest, and stomach lining (mesothelioma)	Used in insulation; may be a contaminant of talc; textile work
Leather	Nasal cavity and sinuses; bladder	Leather and shoe work
Wood	Nasal cavity and sinuses	Woodwork
Chromium	Nasal cavity and sinuses; lung, larynx	Glass, pottery, and linoleum workers; battery makers; textile mill workers
BCME (bi-chloro-methyl ether)	Lung cancer (oat cell type)	Chemical reaction workers; can also be formed spontaneously from formaldehyde and hydrochloric acid (and similar reactions). Traces have been found in permanent-press textile operations.

Aniline dye derivatives	Bladder	Dye manufacturing and use; rubber industry, textile dyeing; paint manufacturing; laboratory work
Auramine		
Benzidine		
β—naphthylamine magenta		
4—aminodiphenyl		
4—nitrodiphenyl		
Vinyl chloride	Liver (angiosarcoma)	Plastics workers and processors
Benzene	Leukemia	Often found as impurity in toluene; rubber cement; sometimes dyestuffs solvent
Carbon tetrachloride	Liver	Dry cleaning
Trichloroethylene†	Liver	Widely used metal degreaser and solvent
Nitrosamines	Lung	Cuttings oils
Polycyclic aromatic hydrocarbons	Lung; skin; scrotum, intestines; pancreas	Contact with oils and waxes; textile weaving
Ionizing radiation	Skin; leukemia	Medical X-ray technologists; dental technicians working with dentures
Radon		
Uranium		
X-ray		
Ultraviolet radiation	Skin	Outdoors workers at risk, especially if working with photosensitizing agents like coal tar pitch

C. METALS

Heavy metals can have a range of effects, some even in trace amounts. Some like arsenic and cadmium are often present as contaminants in other metals.

Cadmium

Extremely toxic; can cause severe kidney damage, cancer, male sterility, and lung damage when inhaled.

Chromium salts	Potent skin allergen. Can also be irritating to nose and throat, and can actually eat through the nasal septum, separating the two parts of the nose. Can cause lung cancer.*
Cobalt	Produces allergic skin reactions and may also produce an asthmatic-type lung response. Compounds of cobalt are toxic when ingested, causing severe stomach pain and weakness in the arms and legs. Recovery is complete. The OSHA standard is probably not protective enough.
Lead	Affects blood-forming tissues and can lead to anemia. Also affects nervous system. Long-term over-exposure is thought to lead to kidney disease and high blood pressure. Blood tests, called ZPP's, should be regularly administered to determine biological effects on blood system, as well as air tests to determine and minimize air levels.
D. IRRITATING GASES AND TOXIC DUST	See Table 20.
E. SKIN ALLERGENS	See Table 18.

* See Part B—Cancer-causing Substances in the Workplace.
† In animals.

NOTES AND BIBLIOGRAPHY

NOTES

Chapter 1: Bound by Conception

1. U. S. Department of Labor Women's Bureau, *1975 Handbook on Women Workers,* p. 10.
2. Ivy Pinchbeck, *Women Workers and the Industrial Revolution, 1750–1850,* chaps. 1–5.
3. Dorothy George, *London Life in the Eighteenth Century,* pp. 168–69.
4. J. Ruskin, "Of Queens' Gardens," *Sesame and Lilies* (1865), in J. A. Banks and Olive Banks, *Feminism and Family Planning,* p. 69.
5. S. A. Sewall, *Women and the Times We Live In,* 2d. ed. (1869), in Banks and Banks, *Feminism,* p. 61.
6. Ann Oakley, *Women's Work: The Housewife Past and Present,* p. 7.
7. Betty Friedan, *The Feminine Mystique,* pp. 224–46.
8. Alva Myrdal and Viola Klein, *Women's Two Roles,* 2d. ed., p. 7.
9. Nathan Mantel and William Haenszel, "Statistical Aspects of the Analysis of Data from Retrospective Studies of Disease," *Journal of the National Cancer Institute* 22 (Apr. 1959): 719–48.
10. Metropolitan Life Insurance Co., *Statistical Bulletin* 55 (Aug. 1974), p. 3.
11. Meyer Friedman and Ray Rosenman, *Type A Behavior Pattern and Your Heart,* p. 62.
12. Robert D. Caplan, Sidney Cobb, John R. P. French, Jr., R. Van Harrison, and S. R. Pinneau, Jr., *Job Demands and Worker*

Health: Main Effects and Occupational Differences (Washington, D. C.: NIOSH, Apr. 1975).

13. Robert B. Sleight et al., *Problems in Occupational Safety and Health: A Critical Review of Select Worker Physical and Psychological Factors* 1 (Cincinnati, Ohio: NIOSH, Nov. 1974), p. C1–C58.

14. *New York Reporter* (White Plains), Feb. 10, 1926, in *Labor Legislation for Women*, Women's Bureau Bulletin no. 66 (Washington, D. C., 1929), p. 100.

15. Testimony of Mrs. Clarence M. Smith, at hearing before the New York State Industrial Survey Commission, Nov. 8, 1926, p. 935.

16. Elizabeth Brandeis, in John R. Commons et al., *History of Labor in the U. S.* 1, 3 vols. (New York: Macmillan, 1918), p. 462.

17. Ibid., p. 463.

18. Muller v. Oregon, 208 U. S. 412 (1908).

19. U. S. Department of Labor Women's Bureau, *Protective Legislation,* Women's Bureau Bulletin no. 66 (Washington, D. C., 1929).

Chapter 2: Work, Stress, and Health

1. A good reference understandable to laymen is Hans Selye, *Stress of Life.*

2. *Work in America,* p. 58.

3. University of Michigan Survey Research Center, *Survey of Working Conditions.*

4. Women's Bureau, *1975 Handbook on Women Workers,* p. 92.

5. U. S. Department of Labor Women's Bureau, *The Economic Role of Women* (Washington, D. C., 1973), p. 109.

6. J. Hedgers and S. Bemis, "Sex Stereotyping: Its Decline in Skilled Trades," *Monthly Labor Review,* pp. 14–22.

7. Charles Speiser, syndicated column in *AFSCME Newsletter* (New York, 1976).

Chapter 3: Health Hazards on the Job

1. *Proceedings of the Conference on Women and the Workplace* (Washington, D. C.: Society for Occupational and Environmental Health, June 1976).

2. Vilma R. Hunt, *The Health of Women at Work.*

3. U. S. Department of Labor Women's Bureau, *Women Workers in Expanding Wartime Industries,* Women's Bureau Bulletin no. 197 (Washington, D. C., 1943), p. 28.

4. U. S. Department of Labor Women's Bureau, *State Reporting of Occupational Disease,* Women's Bureau Bulletin no. 114 (Washington, D. C., 1934), pp. 17–18.

5. A. W. Diddle, "Gravid Women at Work," *Journal of Occupational Medicine* 12 (Jan. 1970): 10–15.

6. Victoria Brown, *Uncommon Lives of Common Women,* p. 724.

7. Paul Brodeur, "Annals of Chemistry: A Compelling Intuition," *The New Yorker,* Nov. 24, 1975, pp. 122–49.

8. A source of current lighting standards is the American National Standards Institute, 1430 Broadway, New York, New York 10018. Stellman and Daum, *Work Is Dangerous to Your Health,* also lists standards.

9. Doris Baldwin, "Caution: Office Zone," *Job Safety and Health,* Feb. 1976, pp. 5–12.

10. Dorothy Richardson, "The Long Day," in *Women at Work,* p. 241.

11. *Encyclopedia of Occupational Health and Safety,* p. 764.

12. See *Work Is Dangerous to Your Health* and other general references in the Bibliography.

13. B. Drummond Ayres, Jr., "Cotton Mills Reset Cost of Curbing Dust," *The New York Times,* May 15, 1977, p. 21.

Chapter 4: Work, Reproduction, and Health

1. Turner v. Board of Review, Department of Employment Security, 531 Pacific 2d. 870 (Utah Supreme Court, 1975).

2. U. S. Department of Health, Education and Welfare, *Employment During Pregnancy: Legitimate Live Births, United States, 1963* (Washington, D. C.: National Center for Health Statistics, 1968).

3. A Stewart, "A Note on the Obstetric Effects of Work During Pregnancy," *British Journal of Preventive Medicine* 9 (1955): 156–61.

4. Vilma R. Hunt, *Occupational Health Problems of Pregnant Women* (Washington, D. C.: U. S. Department of Health, Education and Welfare, 1975).

5. Center for Disease Control, *The Health Consequences of Smoking: A Reference Edition* (Washington, D. C.: U. S. Department of Health, Education and Welfare, 1976), pp. 413–63.

Chapter 5: Social Diseases ... Social Cures

1. Elise Boulding, "Familial Constraints on Women's Work Roles," *SIGNS—Journal of Women in Culture and Society,* p. 105.
2. Minutes of the 1975 meeting of the Environmental Health Committee of the Lead Association, Inc., Sept. 9, 1974.
3. Testimony of Olga M. Madar, president of the Coalition of Labor Union Women (CLUW) on behalf of CLUW on the Occupational Safety and Health Administration's proposed lead standard, Mar. 11, 1977.
4. U. S. Department of Labor Women's Bureau, *The Industrial Nurse and the Woman Worker* (Washington, D. C.: U. S. Department of Labor, 1944).
5. R. Zielhuis and A. Wibówo, "Susceptibility of Adult Females to Lead," *Proceedings of the Second International Workshop on Occupational Exposure to Lead* (Amsterdam, 1976).
6. T. Oliver, *Diseases of Occupation* (New York: Dutton, 1916).
7. Anna Baettjer, *Women in Industry,* pp. 147–49.
8. W. Rom, "Effects of Lead on the Female and Reproduction: A Review," *The Mount Sinai Journal of Medicine* 43, no. 5 (1976): 542–52.
9. Elizabeth Cady Stanton, *Eighty Years and More: Reminiscences 1815–1897,* p. 79.
10. Susan Lynn Vorchheimer v. School District of Philadelphia, 532 Federal 2d. 880 (3d. Cir. 1976).
11. Marilyn Heins, Sue Smock, Jennifer Jacobs, and Margaret Stein, "Productivity of Women Physicians," *Journal of the American Medical Association* 236, no. 17 (1961–1964).
12. Ann Crittenden, "Women and Power—A Status Report," *The New York Times* Business Section, May 3, 1977, p. 1.
13. Women's Bureau, *The Economic Role of Women.*

BIBLIOGRAPHY

For additional helpful bibliographic references, the reader is referred to:

Women's Health

Boston Women's Health Book Collective. *Our Bodies, Ourselves: A Book by and for Women.* New York: Simon & Schuster, 1976.

Housework and Women's Studies

The Feminist Press, Box 334, Old Westbury, New York 11568.

Oakley, Ann. *Woman's Work: The Housewife Past and Present.* New York: Pantheon, 1974.

Health and Safety

Ashford, Nicholas A. *Crisis in the Workplace: Occupational Disease and Injury.* Cambridge, Mass.: MIT Press, 1976.

National Institute of Occupational Safety and Health, 5600 Fishers Lane, Rockville, Maryland 20857.

Urban Planning Aid, 2 Park Square, Boston, Massachusetts 02116.

This selected bibliography consists of some of the references that were useful in the writing of this book.

Women's Health

Assali, Nicholas, ed. *Pathophysiology of Gestation.* New York: Academic Press, 1972.

Baettjer, Anna. *Women in Industry: Their Health and Efficiency.* New York: Saunders, 1946.

Boston Women's Health Book Collective. *Our Bodies, Ourselves: A Book by and for Women.* New York: Simon & Schuster, 1976.

Cromwell, Phyllis, ed. *Women and Mental Health: A Bibliography.* Washington, D. C.: U. S. National Institute of Mental Health, 1974.

Ehrenreich, Barbara, and English, Deirdre. *Complaints and Disorders.* New York: The Feminist Press, 1973. Available from The Feminist Press, Box 334, Old Westbury, New York 11568. ($1.50).

———. *Witches, Midwives, and Nurses: A History of Women Healers.* New York: The Feminist Press, 1973. Available from The Feminist Press, Box 334, Old Westbury, New York 11568. ($1.50).

Hricko, Andrea, with Brunt, Melanie. *Working for Your Life: A Woman's Guide to Job Health Hazards.* Berkeley: Labor Occupational Health Program/Health Research Group, 1976. Available from LOHP, Center for Labor Research and Education, University of California, Berkeley, California 94720.

Hunt, Vilma R. *The Health of Women at Work.* Evanston, Ill.: Program on Women, 1977. Available from Program on Women, 619 Emerson Street, Evanston, Illinois 60201.

———. *Occupational Health Problems of Pregnant Women* SA–5304–75. Washington, D. C.: U. S. Department of Health, Education and Welfare, 1975.

Williams, P. L., and Wendell-Smith, C. P. *Basic Human Embryology*. 2d ed. New York: J. B. Lippincott, 1969.

General and Occupational Health

American Conference of Governmental Hygienists. *Air Sampling Instruments for Evaluation of Atmospheric Contaminants*. 4th ed. Cincinnati, Ohio: American Conference of Governmental Hygienists, 1972. Available from American Conference of Governmental Hygienists, P. O. Box 1937, Cincinnati, Ohio 45201. ($12.50).

Ashford, Nicholas A. *Crisis in the Workplace: Occupational Disease and Injury*. Cambridge, Mass.: MIT Press, 1976.

Brodeur, Paul. *Asbestos and Enzymes*. New York: Ballantine Books, 1972.

———. *Expendable Americans*. New York: Viking Press, 1974.

Browning, Ethel. *Toxicity and Metabolism of Industrial Solvents*. Amsterdam: Elseview, 1965.

———. *Toxicity of Industrial Metals*. 2d ed. London: Butterworth & Co. Ltd., 1969.

Edholm, Otto G. *Biology of Work*. World University Library Series. New York: McGraw-Hill, 1967.

Encyclopedia of Occupational Health and Safety. Geneva: International Labour Office, 1971.

Friedman, Meyer, and Rosenman, Ray. *Type A Behavior Pattern and Your Heart*. New York: Alfred A. Knopf, 1974.

Gleason, Marion N., Gosselin, R. E., and Hodge, H. C. *Clinical Toxicology of Commercial Products*. 3d ed. Baltimore: Williams & Wilkins Co., 1969.

Hamilton, Alice, and Hardy, Harriet. *Industrial Toxicology*. 3d ed. Acton, Mass.: Publishing Sciences Group, 1974.

Hunter, Donald. *The Diseases of Occupations*. 5th ed. Boston: Little, Brown: 1974.

International Occupational Safety and Health Information Centre (CIS). *Noise in Industry*. Information Sheet No. 17. Geneva: International Labour Office, 1968.

Kryter, Karl D. *The Effects of Noise on Man*. New York: Academic Press, 1970. This recent book on noise contains much detailed information, including internationally accepted standards, and is excellent for reference.

Leithead, C. S., and Lind, A. R. *Heat Stress and Heat Disorders*. Philadelphia: Davis, 1964.

Mancuso, Thomas. *Help for the Working Wounded*. Washington, D. C.: International Association of Machinists, 1976. Available from The Machinist, 909 Machinists Building, Washington, D. C. 20036. ($1.00).

The Merck Index of Chemicals and Drugs. 8th ed. Rahway, N. J.: Merck & Co., 1968.

Mott, Paul E., Mann, Floyd C., McLoughlin, Q., and Warwick, D. *Shift Work.* Ann Arbor, Mich.: University of Michigan Press, 1965.

National Academy of Sciences, National Research Council. *The Effects of Exposure to Low Levels of Ionizing Radiation.* Washington, D. C.: U. S. Government Printing Office, 1972.

National Institutes for Occupational Safety and Health. *The Industrial Environment—Its Evaluation and Control.* Washington, D. C.: U. S. Department of Health, Education and Welfare, 1973.

Olishifski, Julian, and McElroy, Frank E., eds. *Fundamentals of Industrial Hygiene.* Chicago: National Safety Council, 1971.

Page, Joseph A., and O'Brien, Mary-Win. *Bitter Wages.* New York: Grossman, 1973.

Patty, Frank A., ed. *Industrial Hygiene and Toxicology.* 2d ed. *Toxicology,* vol. 2. New York: Interscience Publishers, 1963.

Rothman, Harry. *Murderous Providence: A Study of Pollution in Industrial Societies.* Indianapolis: Bobbs-Merrill Co., 1972.

Sax, N. Irving, et al. *Dangerous Properties of Industrial Materials.* 3d ed. New York: Reinhold, 1968.

Selye, Hans. *The Stress of Life.* New York: McGraw-Hill, 1956.

Stellman, Jeanne M., and Daum, Susan M. *Work Is Dangerous to Your Health.* New York: Pantheon, 1973.

U. S. Department of Health, Education and Welfare. There are many available booklets. Request publications list.

———. *The Health Consequences of Smoking—A Reference Edition.* Atlanta, Georgia: U. S. Department of Health, Education and Welfare, 1976.

———. National Institutes for Occupational Safety and Health. The various criteria documents for exposure standards to various conditions are extremely helpful.

U. S. Department of Labor. Occupational Health and Safety Administration. *General Industry Standards.* Washington, D. C.: U. S. Department of Labor, 1976.

University of Michigan Survey Research Center. *Survey of Working Conditions.* Washington, D. C.: U. S. Department of Labor, Employment Standards Division, 1971.

Wallick, Franklin. *The American Worker: An Endangered Species.* New York: Ballantine, 1972.

Wintrobe, M. M., et al., eds. *Harrison's Principles of Internal Medicine.* 6th ed. 2 vols. New York: McGraw-Hill, 1970.

Zenz, Carl, ed. *Occupational Medicine: Principles & Practical Applications.* Chicago: Yearbook Medical Publishers, 1975.

General References on Women

Babcock, Barbara A., et al. *Sex Discrimination and the Law: Causes and Remedies.* Boston: Little, Brown, 1974.

Banks, J. A., and Banks, Olive. *Feminism and Family Planning.* New York: Schocken, 1964.

Baxandell, Roslyn, Gordon, Linda, and Reverby, Susan, eds. *America's Working Woman: A Documentary History—1600 to the Present.* New York: Vintage, 1976.

Brown, Victoria. *Uncommon Lives of Common Women.* Madison, Wisc.: Wisconsin Feminist Project Fund, Inc., 1975. Available from Wisconsin Feminist Project Fund, Inc., P. O. Box 1291, Madison, Wisconsin 53703.

Clark, Alice. *Working Life of Women in the 17th Century.* London: Frank Cass & Co. Ltd., 1968.

Commons, John R., et al. *History of Labor in the U. S.* 3 vols. New York: Macmillan, 1918.

Cook, Alice H. *The Working Mother—A Survey of Problems and Programs in Nine Countries.* New York: NYS School of Industrial and Labor Relations, Cornell University, 1975.

Crozier, Michel. *The World of the Office Worker.* New York: Schocken, 1973.

Cushman, Robert F. *Cases on Constitutional Law.* 4th ed. New Jersey: Prentice Hall, 1975.

Davies, Ross. *Women and Work.* London: Arrow, 1975.

Epstein, Cynthia Fuchs. *Woman's Place: Options and Limits in Professional Careers.* Berkeley: University of California Press, 1971.

Friedan, Betty. *The Feminist Mystique.* New York: Dell, 1963.

George, Dorothy. *London Life in the Eighteenth Century.* New York: Alfred A. Knopf, 1925.

Holcombe, Lee. *Victorian Ladies at Work.* New York: Archon, 1973.

Jephcott, Pearl. *Married Women Working.* London: George Allen Unwin, Ltd., 1962.

Klein, Viola. *Britain's Married Women Workers.* New York: Humanities Press, 1965.

———. *Women Workers.* Paris: OECD, 1965.

Laws, Judith Long. "Work Aspirations of Women: False Leads & New

Starts." *SIGNS—Journal of Women in Culture and Society* 1 (Spring 1976—Supplement, Part 2).

Monthly Labor Review 97 (May 1974).

Myrdal, Alva, and Klein, Viola. *Women's Two Roles*. 2d. ed. London: Routledge & Kegan Paul Ltd., 1968.

National Manpower Council. *Womanpower*. Washington, D. C.: National Manpower Council, 1957.

Oakley, Ann. *The Sociology of Housework*. New York: Pantheon, 1974.

———. *Woman's Work: The Housewife Past and Present*. New York: Pantheon, 1974.

O'Neill, William. *Women at Work*. New York: Quadrangle/The New York Times Book Co., 1972.

Pinchbeck, Ivy. *Women Workers and the Industrial Revolution 1750–1850*. London: Frank Cass & Co. Ltd., 1969.

Ross, Heather L., and Sawhill, Isabel V. *Time of Transition: The Growth of Families Headed by Women*. Washington, D. C.: The Urban Institute, 1975.

Rowbotham, Sheila. *Women, Resistance and Revolution*. New York: Pantheon, 1973.

———. *Hidden from History: Rediscovering Women in History from the 17th Century to the Present*. New York: Pantheon, 1974.

Seifer, Nancy. *Absent from the Majority: Working Class Women in America*. New York: American Jewish Committee, 1973.

SIGNS—Journal of Women in Culture and Society 1 (Spring 1976–Supplement, Part 2).

Smuts, Robert W. *Women and Work in America*. New York: Schocken, 1971.

Stanton, Elizabeth Cady. *Eighty Years and More—Reminiscences 1815–1897*. New York: Schocken, 1971.

Stone, Katherine. *Handbook for OCAW Women*. Denver: Oil, Chemical and Atomic Workers International Union, 1973. Available from Oil, Chemical and Atomic Workers International Union, P. O. Box 2812, Denver, Colorado 80201.

U. S. Bureau of the Census. *1970 Census of Population Characteristics of the Population*. Washington, D. C.: U. S. Bureau of the Census, 1970.

———. *16th Census: Population Comparative Statistics for the United States, 1870–1940*. Washington, D. C.: U. S. Bureau of the Census, 1943.

U. S. Department of Labor Women's Bureau. *1975 Handbook on

Women Workers. Women's Bureau Bulletin no. 297. Washington, D. C.: U. S. Department of Labor, 1975.

————. Women's Bureau Bulletins. Beginning in 1918, these bulletins are an excellent source of occupational health information, demographic data, and social commentary on women workers.

Vanek, Joann. "Time Spent in Housework." *Scientific American* 231 (Nov. 1974): 116–20.

Wertheimer, Barbara Mayer. *We Were There: The Story of Working Women in America.* New York: Pantheon, 1977.

"Women and the Law." 5 Valparaiso University Law Review 203, 488 (1971).

Work in America. Report of a special task force to the Secretary of Health, Education and Welfare. Cambridge, Mass: MIT Press, 1973.

INDEX

ABOUT THE AUTHOR

Jeanne Mager Stellman, author of *Work Is Dangerous to Your Health* (with Susan M. Daum, M.D.), earned a Ph.D. in physical chemistry. She is Chief of the Division of Occupational Health and Toxicology of the American Health Foundation in New York City and Clinical Associate Professor of Research Medicine, School of Medicine, the University of Pennsylvania.